SIRTFOOD DIET RECIPES

A Beginner's Step-By-Step Guide to Rapid Weight Loss, Burning Fat, and Healthy Living – Enjoy Over 100 Delicious Recipes and Discover a Meal Plan to Lose Weight in 7 Days!

MELANIE STEVIE

TABLE OF CONTENTS

INTRODUCTION

While new diets emerge every day, the Sirtfood Diet is the latest diet trend. The main goal of this diet is to shed a considerable amount of weight within a span of three weeks. Not only that, but the Sirtfood Diet can help in dealing with various chronic problems such as reduction of inflammation. This diet is considered to be a revolutionary diet plan that functions by turning on the sirtuins or skinny genes. Sirtuins are a special group of proteins that are essential for losing weight. This group of proteins can help in other body functions such as improving body metabolism, prevention of cancer, improvement of lifespan, and others.

This book is all about the various aspects of the Sirtfood Diet, along with several tasty meal recipes that will be making your weight loss journey more exciting. After you complete all the phases of the diet, you can continue including several types of sirtfoods in your daily diet. This will help you keep the weight off. According to the creators of the Sirtfood Diet, the diet plan can readily help in shedding extra pounds while maintaining your muscle mass at the same time. You will also find a 7-day meal plan at the end of this book.

There are plenty of books on this subject on the market, thanks again for choosing this one! Every effort was made to ensure it is full of as much useful information as possible. Thanks again for taking the time to read this book. Be sure to leave a short review. If you enjoy it, I'd really love to hear your thoughts

CHAPTER 1:
THE SIRTFOOD DIET

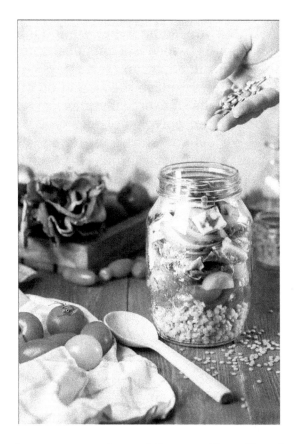

Sirtfood Diet is a new member of the trending diet plans that have been quite popular for the last few years. This diet plan was developed by two nutritionists from the United Kingdom. During the initial days of the diet plan, it was marketed as being the 'revolutionary diet plan.' The primary goal of this diet is to restrict the consumption of calories that will ultimately lead to weight loss. It functions by the activation of the skinny genes, and if you want to know more about it, read on.

What is the Sirt Diet?

The Sirt Diet is all about the burning of excess body fat that can otherwise disturb the state of your health. Unlike other types of diets, the Sirt Diet focuses on weight loss without experiencing starvation or malnutrition. Skinny genes can be activated by fasting and exercising. There are some types of food items that are composed of polyphenols (which is a chemical compound). When such food items are consumed, it can exert stress on the cells of the body. This will ultimately result in the formation of the genes that can follow the end-results of exercising and fasting. Some of the food items that are rich in polyphenols are green tea, coffee, red wine, kale, and so on. As you start consuming such food items, sirtuins are released that imparts various effects on the body. Some of the effects of sirtuins are mood swings, improvement of the metabolic rate, aging, etc.

Although this diet has a wide range of benefits, it is very restrictive in nature for certain food items along with the intake of calories. So, it can be said that the diet plan might turn out to be complex for certain people, and you will have to put in some effort if you want to make it a habit.

Sirtuins

Sirtuins are a group of special proteins that can perform deacetylase activities. They come with various types of enzymes that can perform several functions in improving cell life and also for the prevention of aging. Sirtuins consume NAD+ or nicotinamide-adenine-dinucleotide as they cannot function without their presence. Several studies have been conducted regarding sirtuins that proved their importance in human bodies. The first sirtuin was discovered by Dr. Amar Jit Singh Klar in the 1970s. It was named SIR2. It is a gene that is responsible for controlling the mating process of yeast cells. In was during the 1990s when some researchers discovered cells that are of homologous nature to the SIR2. These cells were discovered in worms and fruit flies. These cells came to be known as the sirtuins.

There are some specific food items that can activate sirtuins. They are also known as SIRT that can be found in human bodies. They are seven in number that ranges from SIRT1 to SIRT7. There are several benefits that have been proved by various researchers regarding these food items. Such food items come with the power of mimicking the overall benefits of restriction of calories along with fasting as they can easily activate the sirtuins. Some other benefits of sirtuins are turning on and off the genes, preventing the cells from aging, reduction of inflammation, and others. All those food items that can turn on the sirtuins are called sirtfoods.

Benefits of the Diet

There are various benefits related to this diet.

- **Lose excess body weight:** This diet plan is well known for the shedding of extra body weight. It can also help in several other benefits for the body as it comes with anti-inflammatory properties. The diet depends mainly on the intake of various types of juices that are rich in minerals and vitamins. However, as it is mainly based on juices, it lacks the presence of essential fiber from the whole fruits and veggies.

- **Gain lean muscle mass:** Gaining lean muscle while burning fat might not seem that easy. However, it is possible with the Sirtfood Diet. The best thing about this diet is that it does not affect the muscle mass while burning fat, which is the case with other types of diets. The developers of this diet claimed that it is possible to lose about 3 kgs or 7 pounds during the first phase of the diet. The activated SIRT genes help a lot in preserving the lean muscle mass and also burn body fat at the same time. Also, the activated SIRT genes help in boosting the recovery and growth of muscles. This diet plan can easily improve the overall functioning of the muscles.

- **Prevents cancer:** Some studies claim that the Sirtfood Diet can also help in preventing the onset of cancer. SIRT1 genes help in the reduction of tumors. The diet is well known for reduction of inflammation. In fact, sirtfoods are also loaded with antioxidants that can help in treating tumors. That is the reason why it is believed to prevent the onset of cancer. However, it lacks enough evidence for proving this claim.

- **Treats Alzheimer's disease:** People suffering from Alzheimer's disease can be treated with the help of this diet. It can also help in improving the sensitivity to insulin.

Phases of Sirtfood Diet

The diet has been divided into two main phases that last for a span of three weeks. After you complete the phases of the diet, you can continue including sirtfoods in your daily diet for maintaining the lost weight. But, you will need to follow the two phases of the diet properly, and you will need to keep a check on the same.

The diet depends mainly on the essential green juice that plays a very important role in the diet plan. You will need to consume this juice at least three times a day.

- **Phase one:** The first phase of the diet will last for one week. The main aim of this week is to restrict the intake of calories. Restriction of calories can be done easily by giving up on the high carb foods and just focus on the green juice. This form of change in the diet will be helping you to jump-start the program of losing weight. It is true that the change is drastic in nature, and thus it has claimed that you will shed 3 kgs or 7 pounds in the first phase only. The intake of calories needs to be restricted to 1000 calories for the first three days. From the fourth day of the week, the calorie intake can be increased by 500 only. The meal plan will include three juices and one meal during the first three days. From the fourth day, you can include one more meal and remove one juice.

- **Phase two or Maintenance phase:** This is the last phase of the Sirtfood Diet and is often known as the **Maintenance phase.** It will last for two weeks. The aim of this phase is to continue with the diet of the first phase with proper restriction of calories. This phase needs to be properly maintained, since there is a chance of gaining back the lost weight during this time. You can choose your meals from the recipes that will be mentioned in the upcoming chapters.

Sirtfoods

There are various food items that can be included in the diet plan, and I have made a list of them below.

Arugula

This is regarded as the most important sirtfood veggie, and that is why tops the list. It is essential for keeping a proper check on your weight and comes with other healthy properties as well. It is very low in calories. A hundred grams of arugula contains only about 25 calories. It is rich in fiber content and can be consumed with salads as well. It comes with vitamins A, C, K, and folate.

Celery

Celery stalks are rich in dietary fibers and can aid in losing weight. One stalk of celery comes with about 10 calories. It can help in dealing with dehydration as it consists of a great number of electrolytes along with water.

Cocoa

Cocoa is beneficial for metabolizing body fat in a better way. It can help in preventing inflammation and can also aid in the process of digestion. It also helps in detoxification of the body as it comes with antioxidants of various types, such as flavonoids. Cocoa can also help in maintaining the level of blood sugar.

Red Wine

Red wine comes with a polyphenol known as resveratrol that can help in losing weight. Consumption of red wine in moderate quantities can help in reducing the risk of strokes and heart attacks.

Green Tea
Often considered as the healthiest beverage on the planet, green tea can help in shedding the extra pounds. It comes loaded with antioxidants along with several other plant compounds. The most important compound that is present in green tea is caffeine. Caffeine is a stimulant that helps in the burning of fat.

Kale
With one cup of raw kale, you can provide your body with about 2.4 grams of dietary fibers. Dietary fibers are very important for the reduction of hunger. This vegetable is rich in vitamins, minerals, and proteins. In fact, it comes with a great amount of calcium.

Some other sirtfoods include buckwheat, caper, chilies, medjool dates, garlic, parsley, red onion, red endive, olive oil, ginger, and turmeric.

CHAPTER 2:
RECIPES FOR SMOOTHIES
AND JUICES

Sirtfood Diet is all about smoothies and juices. The majority of the diet plan will include smoothies and juices, as it is the secret to weight loss. So, this chapter is all about some of the tastiest sirtfood smoothies and juices that will make your diet journey a lot more exciting.

Sirtfood Green Juice

Total Prep & Cooking Time: 3 minutes
Yields: 1 serving
Nutrition Facts: Calories: 91 | Carbs: 24g | Protein: 2.7g | Fat: 0g |Fiber: 5.3g

Ingredients:

- Five grams parsley
- Eighty-five grams kale
- One green apple (large)
- Two celery stalks
- One small lemon (juiced)
- Forty grams of arugula (rocket variety)
- Half centimeter ginger
- Half tbsp. Matcha green tea powder

Method:

1. Cut down all the listed ingredients except for the lemon and green tea into small pieces. Cutting the ingredients into small pieces will help you to put them into the juicer. In case you want to juice each of the ingredients separately, you can do that as well.

2. Add lemon juice to the prepared juice from the top and give it a stir. You can squeeze the lemon with your hand also.
3. Take some of the prepared juice in a glass and add matcha green tea to it. Stir the juice properly. Add the remaining juice to the glass and stir it again.
4. Drink the prepared juice straight away.

Notes:

You can prepare the juice at large quantities at once and store it in the freezer for three days. So, just prepare it once a day, and you can enjoy the goodness of the green juice for the next three days.

Pineapple Kale Smoothie

Total Prep & Cooking Time: 5 minutes
Yields: 2 servings
Nutrition Facts: Calories: 190 | Carbs: 25g | Protein: 7.8g | Fat: 1g
|Fiber: 4.1g

Ingredients:

- Two cups of kale leaves (lightly packed, remove the stems)
- One cup unsweetened almond milk (vanilla or any other type of milk)
- One medium-sized banana (frozen, chopped in chunks)
- One cup plain yogurt (Greek)
- One-third cup pineapple chunks (frozen)
- One and a half tbsps. peanut butter
- 2 – 3 tbsps. honey

Method:

1. Start by placing all the listed ingredients in a blender in this order- kale, banana, yogurt, almond milk, peanut butter, pineapple, and honey. Blend the ingredients properly until smooth and frothy.
2. In case you want to reduce the consistency of the smoothie, you can add more almond milk to reach the consistency you want.
3. Pour the smoothie into glasses and enjoy!

Notes:

- In case you are using a blender of low power, you can blend the ingredients one by one and then give all the ingredients a whirl.
- You can add ice cubes to the smoothie for making the smoothie thick and chilled.
- The leftover smoothie can be stored in the freezer for two days.

Blueberry Pie Smoothie

Total Prep & Cooking Time: 5 minutes
Yields: 1 serving
Nutrition Facts: Calories: 190 | Carbs: 36g | Protein: 18g | Fat: 3g
|Fiber: 6.2g

Ingredients:

- Half cup blueberries (frozen)
- One medium-sized banana (frozen, chopped)
- One cup plain yogurt (non-fat)
- Half tbsp. almond butter
- Two tbsps. rolled oats
- One cup of almond milk (unsweetened)
- One tsp. vanilla extract
- Half tsp. cinnamon (ground)
- Half scoop vanilla protein powder (optional)
- Two tsps. maple syrup (optional)

Method:

1. Place yogurt, oats, blueberries, banana, almond butter, cinnamon, vanilla, and protein powder (optional) in a high-speed blender. Blend the ingredients until creamy and smooth.
2. In case the smoothie is thick, you can add more almond milk to the smoothie and blend.
3. Add maple syrup to it after tasting.
4. Blend the smoothie once more and pour it into a glass.
5. Serve immediately.

Notes:

- In case you do want to use almond milk, you can use milk of any other type.
- Adding cinnamon will not only be adding a spicy taste to the smoothie but will also make it more delicious. Also, it comes with various health benefits such as it helps in controlling blood sugar, helps in boosting brain power, and so on.

Strawberry Smoothie

Total Prep & Cooking Time: Four minutes
Yields: Four Servings
Nutritional Facts: Calories: 90 | Protein: 5g | Fat: 4.2g | Carbs: 18.3g | Fiber: 6.2g

Ingredients:

- One cup strawberries (whole, frozen)
- One cup plain yogurt (Greek, non-fat)
- One tbsp. almond butter
- One tsp. vanilla extract
- Three tsps. honey
- One cup of almond milk (unsweetened)

Method:

1. Start by placing the listed ingredients in a high-speed blender. Blend the ingredients until frothy and creamy.
2. Add honey to the smoothie according to your taste.
3. Pour into smoothie glasses and enjoy.

Notes:

- You can make the smoothie dairy-free by using non-dairy yogurt. In case you want a vegan smoothie, use maple syrup in place of honey. You can leave out yogurt and add a banana for adding creaminess to the smoothie.
- In case you do not have a high-power blender, it will be better if you can blend the strawberries first. You can also slice the strawberries as it will make the blending process faster. You might need to add in more almond milk and stir the blender at times for ensuring proper mixing of the smoothie.
- You can store the leftover smoothie in an airtight jar for two days in the freezer.

Beet Smoothie

Total Prep & Cooking Time: 6 minutes
Yields: 2 Servings
Nutrition Facts: Calories: 92 | Protein: 5.2g | Fat: 1g | Carbs: 18.2g
| Fiber: 4.3g

Ingredients:

- One small-sized beet (peeled, diced)
- Half cup almond milk (unsweetened, milk of your choice)
- One cup blueberries (frozen)
- One-fourth cup pineapple (frozen)
- Half cup plain yogurt (Greek)
- Two tsps. honey (optional)
- Chia seeds (optional)

Method:

1. Start by placing all the ingredients in a blender in this order-beet, blueberries, pineapple, almond milk, and yogurt. You can chop the pineapple into small cubes for making the process of blending easier. Blend the ingredients until smooth.
2. Taste the smoothie and add honey to it according to your taste. Add chia seeds (if using) and blend again.
3. Pour the smoothie in glasses and serve immediately.

Notes:

- If you do not like too much beet in your smoothie, you can reduce its quantity.
- You can also use a mix of berries in place of blueberries.
- You can add one tbsp. of oatmeal to the smoothie for reducing the flavor of beet.
- The leftover smoothie can be stored in the freezer for one day.
- If you are using low power blender, blend the beet first.

Turmeric Berry Smoothie

Total Prep & Cooking Time: 5 minutes
Yields: 2 Servings
Nutrition Facts: Calories: 132 | Protein: 7g | Fat: 3g | Carbs: 25g |
Fiber: 3.2g

Ingredients:

- One-fourth cup almond milk (unsweetened, milk of your choice)
- One cup spinach (about one handful)
- Half cup of Greek yogurt (non-fat, plain)
- One and a half cup of mixed berries (frozen)
- Four tbsps. rolled oats
- Half tsp. ground turmeric
- One-fourth tsp. ginger (ground)
- Three tsps. honey (you can use any other sweetener)

Method:

1. Place the listed ingredients in the blender in this order-spinach, almond milk, yogurt, berries, oats, ginger, turmeric, and honey. Blend all the ingredients until smooth and frothy.
2. Taste the smoothie and add honey if needed according to your taste.
3. Divide the smoothie into glasses and serve.

Notes:
- If you do not have a high power blender, blend yogurt, almond milk, and spinach first. You can add the rest of the ingredients after that.
- This smoothie can help in preventing cold or flu as it contains ginger and turmeric.
- If you do not like the taste of spinach, add more berries for mellowing the taste of spinach.
- The leftover smoothie can be stored in the freezer for one day.

Date and Blueberry Shake

Total Prep & Cooking Time: 10 minutes
Yields: 2 Servings
Nutrition Facts: Calories: 238 | Protein: 4.8g | Fat: 5.9g | Carbs: 52g | Fiber: 7.3g

Ingredients:

- Two medium-sized bananas (frozen, chopped into chunks)
- Four Medjool dates (pitted)
- One and a half cup blueberries (frozen)
- One tbsp. almond butter
- Half tsp. of vanilla extract
- One cup of almond milk (vanilla, unsweetened)
- Half cup ice cubes

Method:

1. Place blueberries, banana, almond butter, dates, almond milk, and vanilla extract in a blender. Blend the ingredients properly until smooth.
2. Add ice cubes to the blender and blend again.
3. Taste the shake and add almond butter to it if you want it to be richer.
4. Blend again.
5. Pour the shake into glasses and enjoy.

Notes:

- Blend half portion of the frozen fruits and almond milk first if you do not have a high power blender. Add the remaining ingredients after that.
- For making the shake thicker, add more ice cubes to it.
- You can add more dates to the shake if you want it sweeter.
- You can store the leftover shake in a container in the fridge for two days.

Avocado Blueberry Banana Smoothie

Total Prep & Cooking Time: Ten minutes
Yields: Two Servings
Nutritional Facts: Calories: 242 | Protein: 7g | Fat: 1.9g | Carbs: 43g
| Fiber: 12g

Ingredients:

- One cup spinach (fresh)
- Half cup vanilla almond milk (unsweetened)
- One small banana (peeled)
- One ripe avocado (peeled, pitted)
- Two and a half cups blueberries (frozen)
- One tbsp. flaxseed meal (ground)
- One tsp. ground cinnamon
- One tbsp. almond butter

Method:

1. Start by placing all the ingredients in a blender in this order-almond milk, banana, spinach, avocado, flaxseed meal, blueberries, and almond butter.
2. Blend the ingredients properly until smooth.
3. Add cinnamon from the top and blend again.
4. Divide the smoothie in glasses and serve.

Notes:

- If you have a high power blender, you can use whole almonds in place of almond butter. It will make sure that the smoothie is smooth.
- In case you want the smoothie to be thick, you can add one cup of ice at the time of blending. For reducing the consistency of the smoothie, add more almond milk.
- You can store the leftover smoothie in an airtight container for three days. Store the container in the freezer.

Mint Avocado Smoothie

Total Prep & Cooking Time: 10 minutes
Yields: 1 Serving
Nutrition Facts: Calories: 178 | Protein: 2.3g | Fat: 9.6g | Carbs: 17g | Fiber: 8.2g

Ingredients:

- One cup spinach leaves (fresh, firmly packed)
- Two bananas (frozen, chopped)
- Three-fourth cup of almond milk (unsweetened)
- One medium-sized avocado
- One-fourth tsp. peppermint extract
- One cup mint leaves (fresh)
- Sweetener of your choice
- One cup whipped cream (optional)
- Dark chocolate (shaved, optional)

Method:

1. Place the listed ingredients in the blender except for the dark chocolate shavings and whipped cream. Blend all the ingredients until smooth and properly combined.
2. Taste the smoothie and add sweetener according to your taste.
3. Divide the smoothie into glasses and top with dark chocolate and whipped cream.
4. Serve immediately.

Notes:

- For the sweetener, you can use liquid stevia, maple syrup, honey, or Truvia.
- This smoothie is a perfect choice for the summer days as it comes loaded with the freshness of mint. It can help in boosting your energy level.
- You can add a few ice cubes to the smoothie at the time of blending if you want the smoothie chilled.
- Almond milk can be replaced with any other type of milk.

Kale Blueberry Smoothie

Total Prep & Cooking Time: 10 minutes
Yields: 1 Serving
Nutrition Facts: Calories: 226 | Protein: 16.3g | Fat: 3.3g | Carbs:
38.6g | Fiber: 7.1g

Ingredients:

- One medium-sized banana
- Half cup kale (fresh, chopped)
- One cup blueberries (frozen or fresh)
- Half cup plain low-fat yogurt
- One scoop of protein powder (any flavor of your choice or unflavored)
- Half tsp. ground cinnamon
- Two cups of ice cubes
- One tbsp. flaxseed meal

Method:

1. Start by placing all the ingredients in a high power blender. Keep blending until smooth. You can add the ice cubes as per the required consistency.
2. Pour the smoothie in a glass and enjoy.

Notes:

- Kale is a great superfood and can provide you with a boost of nutrients. It is rich in vitamins A, C, and K. It can also help in preventing heart diseases and can provide bone health.
- For reducing the consistency of the smoothie, you can add a splash of water at the time of blending.
- The leftover smoothie can be stored in the freezer for one day.
- You can also use a mix of berries in place of blueberries.

Strawberry and Chocolate Smoothie

Total Prep & Cooking Time: 10 minutes
Yields: 2 Serving
Nutrition Facts: Calories: 230 | Protein: 21.2g | Fat: 4.6g | Carbs: 31g | Fiber: 6.9g

Ingredients:

- One cup strawberries (frozen or fresh)
- One cup plain yogurt (low fat)
- One medium-sized ripe banana
- Half cup protein powder
- Two tbsps. of each
  - Flaxseed meal
  - Cocoa powder
- One tsp. ground cinnamon
- Half cup ice cubes
- Half tsp. vanilla extract

Method:
1. Start by placing all the ingredients in a high-speed blender. Keep blending until the smoothie is frothy and smooth.
2. Add ice cubes to the smoothie and blend again.
3. Pour the smoothie in glasses and top with ground cinnamon.
4. Serve immediately.

Notes:
- This smoothie is rich in protein as it consists of cocoa powder, yogurt, and cinnamon.
- It is a great choice for the summer days.
- You can adjust the thickness of the smoothie by adding ice and water.
- If you want the smoothie sweeter, add half tsp. of honey or any other sweetener.
- If you do not have a high power blender, you can crush the ice first with the strawberries and then add the rest of the ingredients.

Espresso Chocolate Smoothie

Total Prep & Cooking Time: 10 minutes
Yields: 1 Serving
Nutrition Facts: Calories: 261 | Protein: 25g | Fat: 3.3g | Carbs: 38.6g | Fiber: 5.2g

Ingredients:

- Two-third cup Greek yogurt (vanilla)
- One cup almond milk (unsweetened, milk of your choice)
- One large banana
- One tbsp. cocoa powder
- Two tsps. instant espresso coffee (you can use any other instant coffee)
- One tsp. vanilla extract
- Two cups of ice cubes

Method:

1. Place the ingredients in a high-speed blender except for the cubes of ice. Blend the ingredients until combined properly and smooth.
2. Add ice cubes according to the required consistency.
3. Serve immediately.

Notes:

- For the best results, add the liquid ingredients to the blender first and then top it with ice cubes.
- If you want the smoothie to be thinner, just skip the ice. For having a thick smoothie, add more cubes of ice.
- This smoothie is a perfect companion for boosting your energy level as it contains coffee that is rich in caffeine.
- You can add choco chips from the top at the time of serving along with some shavings of dark chocolate.

Mint Strawberry Smoothie

Total Prep & Cooking Time: Ten minutes
Yields: 2 Servings
Nutritional Facts: Calories: 270 | Protein: 7g | Fat: 12g | Carbs: 29g
| Fiber: 9.2g

Ingredients:

- One large-sized banana
- One cup strawberries (frozen or fresh)
- One cup of coconut milk (full fat)
- One tsp. vanilla extract
- Two tbsps. flax seed (whole or ground)
- Two tbsps. mint leaves (fresh)
- One cup of ice cubes
- Three tbsps. cocoa powder

Method:

1. Place all the ingredients in the blender except for mint leaves and ice cubes. Blend the smoothie until frothy and smooth.
2. Add ice cubes along with the mint leaves. Give the smoothie a nice whirl.
3. Pour the smoothie in glasses and serve.

Notes:

- For better taste, do not blend the mint leaves completely. Leave them slightly crushed.
- You can replace coconut milk with almond milk as well. You can also use yogurt of any type for making the smoothie creamy and thick. Avocado can also be used if you do not have coconut milk.
- The mint will be adding a fresh aroma to the smoothie and is perfect for the summer days.
- You can add some chunks of dark chocolate at the time of blending for extra flavor.

Berry Banana Smoothie

Total Prep & Cooking Time: 8 minutes
Yields: 1 Serving
Nutrition Facts: Calories: 252 | Protein: 23.5g | Fat: 3g | Carbs: 38.7g | Fiber: 10g

Ingredients:

- One cup of mixed berries (frozen)
- Half cup plain yogurt (Greek)
- One banana
- One scoop protein powder
- One cup of water
- Half tbsp. flaxseed meal
- One tsp. ground cinnamon
- One tsp. ginger (fresh, grated, optional)
- One cup of ice cubes
- Two cups baby spinach (fresh)

Method:

1. Start by placing all the listed ingredients in a blender except for the ice cubes.
2. Blend the ingredients until smooth and frothy.
3. Add the ice cubes and give it a pulse.
4. Pour the smoothie into a glass and enjoy.

Notes:

- Depending on the power of the blender that you are using, you can puree all the ingredients first and then add the ice cubes. If the blender is of high power, you can add all the ingredients along with the ice cubes at once.
- This smoothie is a great source of fiber and thus can help you stay full for a longer period of time.
- You can use protein powder of any flavor.

Berry Ginger Fruit Smoothie

Total Prep & Cooking Time: Twenty minutes
Yields: Two Servings
Nutritional Facts: Calories: 173 | Protein: 8.2g | Fat: 3.6g | Carbs: 36g | Fiber: 10.3g

Ingredients:

- One apple (cored, quartered)
- One large banana (fresh or frozen)
- One cup of mixed berries (frozen)
- Two cups spinach (frozen)
- Twp tbsps. flaxseed meal
- One inch of ginger (sliced)
- Half cup of ice cubes
- One cup of water

Method:

1. Add the listed ingredients in the blender in this order-banana, apple, spinach, berries, ginger, flaxseed meal, and water.
2. Blend the ingredients properly until smooth.
3. Add ice cubes to the blender and give it a pulse.
4. Pour the smoothie into glasses and serve.

Notes:

- Adding ginger to the smoothie will help in adding a zing to the smoothie and will transform the dull smoothie into an exciting one.
- You can replace frozen berries with fresh ones if you want to use a lot of ice cubes. If you do not have ice cubes, you can use frozen berries for making the smoothie creamy and thick.
- Add a splash of water for adjusting the consistency of the smoothie.

Ginger Blueberry Peach Smoothie

Total Prep & Cooking Time: 15 minutes
Yields: 1 Serving
Nutrition Facts: Calories: 192 | Protein: 14g | Fat: 2.8g | Carbs: 37g | Fiber: 7g

Ingredients:

- One cup blueberries
- One fresh peach (halved, remove the pit)
- One large banana
- Two scoops of protein powder (vanilla)
- Two tbsps. ginger (one-inch piece)
- Three tbsps. flaxseed meal
- Half cup of water
- One cup of ice cubes

Method:

1. Pulse all the listed ingredients in a blender except for the ice cubes. Blend until frothy and smooth.
2. Add the ice cubes for adjusting the consistency of the smoothie.
3. Pour the smoothie into two tall glasses and serve.

Notes:

- For making the smoothie thin, add few cubes of ice. For making the smoothie thicker, add more ice cubes.
- Adding ginger to the smoothie will be bringing out the sweetness of the fruits.
- You can use both fresh and frozen blueberries.
- The leftover smoothie can be stored in the freezer for three days. You can make a large batch of the smoothie at once and enjoy it for the next three days.

Mango Blueberry Smoothie

Total Prep & Cooking Time: 10 minutes
Yields: 2 Servings
Nutrition Facts: Calories: 223 | Protein: 16.5g | Fat: 3.3g | Carbs: 49g | Fiber: 8g

Ingredients:

- One cup blueberries (frozen)
- One cup ripe mango (cubed)
- One medium-sized banana
- One lime (peeled)
- One cup plain yogurt (low fat)
- One cup parsley
- Two scoops of protein powder
- One inch ginger root (diced)
- Two tbsps. flaxseed meal
- Two cups of ice cubes
- One cup of water

Method:

1. Take a high-speed blender and start adding all the listed ingredients except for the ice cubes.
2. Blend the ingredients until smooth.
3. Add ice cubes according to the required consistency.
4. Pour the smoothie into two tall glasses and garnish with ripe mangoes from the top.
5. Serve immediately.

Notes:

- This smoothie is packed with protein and nutrients. So, it can provide you with a great supply of energy all day long.

- If you do not have a high power blender, blend the ingredients first. Blend the ice cubes separately and add the same to the smoothie afterward.
- You can use Greek yogurt in place of plain yogurt.
- You can chill the mango cubes before blending for making the smoothie creamy.

Chia Banana Strawberry Mango Smoothie

Total Prep & Cooking Time: 10 minutes
Yields: 2 Servings
Nutrition Facts: Calories: 230 | Protein: 14.3g | Fat: 4.7g | Carbs: 48g | Fiber: 9.7g

Ingredients:

- One large banana
- One cup strawberries (frozen or fresh)
- One ripe mango (pitted, peeled, chopped)
- One cup of yogurt (Greek)
- One tsp. ginger (ground)
- One tbsp. flaxseed meal
- Two cups of ice cubes
- One tsp. ground cinnamon
- Two tsps. chia seeds

Method:

1. Add mango, strawberries, banana, yogurt, ginger, flaxseed meal, and cinnamon in a high power blender.
2. Blend the ingredients at high speed for 40 seconds.
3. Add ice cubes to the blender and give it a pulse.
4. Pour the smoothie into tall glasses and serve with chia seeds from the top.

Notes:

- If you want to use frozen fruits, there is no need to use ice cubes.
- The leftover smoothie can be stored in the freezer for one day.

CHAPTER 3:
RECIPES FOR VEGETABLES

There are various types of vegetables that you can include in your Sirtfood Diet plan. Vegetables are a great source of fiber and thus can help you in staying full for a longer time.

Zucchini Pumpkin Lasagna

Total Prep & Cooking Time: One hour and fifteen minutes
Yields: 6 Servings
Nutrition Facts: Calories: 295 | Protein: 30g | Fat: 15g | Carbs: 30.6g | Fiber: 11.2g

Ingredients:

- Six-hundred grams of butternut pumpkin (sliced thinly)
- Cooking spray (olive oil)
- Two zucchinis (peeled, peel like ribbons)
- One tbsp. olive oil (extra virgin)
- One large onion (chopped finely)
- Four cloves of garlic (crushed)
- Half tsp. cinnamon (ground)
- One tsp. allspice (ground)
- One cup tomatoes (sundried)
- 500 g canned tomatoes (crushed)
- One cup red lentils
- Two tbsps. oregano (fresh, chopped)
- 300 g ricotta
- Half cup parmesan cheese (grated)

Method:

1. Start with preheating the oven at 200 degrees Celsius. Use baking paper for lining two baking sheets.

2. Place pumpkin slices in one layer in the first tray. Spray it with oil. Roast the pumpkin for 10 minutes and keep it aside.
3. Place the zucchini ribbons in a tray and roast it for 5 minutes after spraying with oil.
4. Take a pan and heat oil in it over a medium flame. Add the garlic along with all the spices to the pan. Add tomatoes and lentils to the pan. Cook the mixture for 10 minutes and add three cups of water.
5. Add oregano to the lentil mix.
6. Combine parmesan and ricotta in a bowl and season with salt.
7. Grease a deep baking dish and add pumpkin slices as the base. Top it with lentil and tomato mix and add zucchini ribbons on top of it. Repeat the same with the remaining mixture.
8. Add cheese mixture from the top and cover the dish with a foil.
9. Bake the lasagna for twenty-five minutes. Remove foil cover and bake for another ten minutes.
10. Serve hot.

Peanut, Tofu, and Quinoa Fried Rice

Total Prep & Cooking Time: 40 minutes
Yields: Four Servings
Nutritional Facts: Calories: 300 | Protein: 21g | Fat: 10g | Carbs: 29g | Fiber: 15g

Ingredients:

- 200 grams quinoa (rinsed and drained)
- Two cups of water
- Two tsps. peanut oil
- 300 grams of tofu (firm, cubed)
- One large carrot (peeled, sliced)
- Two stalks of celery (fresh, sliced)
- Two cloves of garlic (crushed)
- One bunch of choy sum (trimmed)
- One cup of green peas
- Two tbsps. tamari sauce
- Two tsps. lime juice
- Two tsps. sambal oelek
- Two tbsps. peanuts (roasted, unsalted, chopped)
- Coriander (for garnishing)

Method:
1. Add water and quinoa in a saucepan. Boil the water. Reduce the flame and cook for 15 minutes or until the quinoa gets tender.
2. Add half of the oil in a skillet over a high flame. Add tofu cubes and fry it for 4 minutes.
3. Add remaining oil to the pan and heat it over a medium flame. Add carrot, onion, along with celery. Fry the mixture for two minutes.
4. Add garlic to the pan along with peas and choy sum.
5. Add tofu along with tamari sauce to the pan. Add quinoa and sambal.
6. Stir fry the mixture for 2 minutes.
7. Serve with coriander and peanuts from the top.

Stuffed Capsicum

Total Prep & Cooking Time: 50 minutes
Yields: 4 Servings
Nutrition Facts: Calories: 232 | Protein: 14.3g | Fat: 6g | Carbs: 22g | Fiber: 13g

Ingredients:
- Four red capsicums (deseeded, halved)
- 500 grams of canned beans (cannellini, rinsed)
- Two large tomatoes (deseeded, chopped)
- One large zucchini (chopped finely)
- Three shallots (sliced thinly)
- 100 grams feta (crumbled)
- One-fourth cup of kalamata olives (finely chopped)
- One-fourth cup parsley (fresh, chopped)
- Two tsps. lemon rind (grated)
- 300 grams grape tomatoes (halved)
- 200 grams rocket arugula
- Two tsps. vinegar (balsamic)

Method:
1. Preheat your oven to 200 degrees Celsius. Use parchment paper for lining a baking tray.
2. Place the halved capsicums with the cut side up on the tray. Roast the capsicums for about 10 minutes.
3. Take a large bowl and add beans, tomatoes, shallots, zucchini, parsley, olives, feta, along with lemon rind. Toss the ingredients properly. Add pepper for seasoning.
4. Drain out the liquid from the capsicum, if any. Divide the prepared mixture among the roasted capsicums.
5. Bake the capsicums for about 20 minutes or until they get soft.
6. Add grape tomatoes along with arugula in a bowl. Add vinegar to the bowl and toss.
7. Serve the cooked capsicum with tomato and arugula salad.

Notes:

You can use lemon juice in place of vinegar with a little bit of salt.

Zucchini Slice

Total Prep & Cooking Time: 50 minutes
Yields: 6 Servings
Nutrition Facts: Calories: 190 | Protein: 14g | Fat: 8.2g | Carbs: 10.2g | Fiber: 7.2g

Ingredients:

- Two tsps. olive oil (extra virgin)
- One large onion (chopped finely)
- Two cloves of garlic (crushed)
- Two large carrots (trimmed, grated)
- 200 grams kale (fresh, chopped)
- 10 eggs
- 100 grams of ricotta cheese
- Four zucchinis (grated, squeeze out the excess moisture)
- Two tbsps. parsley (fresh, chopped)
- 200 grams quinoa (cooked)
- 200 grams of grape tomatoes (halved)

Method:

1. Preheat your over at 180 degrees Celsius. Take a baking pan and spray it with oil. Line the pan with baking paper.
2. Take a skillet and add oil to it over a medium flame. Add onions to the oil and cook it for 5 minutes. Stir the onion occasionally.
3. Add carrot and garlic to the onion and cook for one more minute.
4. Add kale to the skillet and cook until it wilts. Season with salt and pepper and give it a stir.
5. Take a bowl and whisk together ricotta and eggs. Add the cooked veggies to the mixture along with parsley, zucchini, and quinoa.
6. Give the mixture a nice stir.
7. Add the zucchini mixture to the prepared pan and top it with tomatoes.

8. Bake it for about thirty minutes. Make sure it is golden in color.
9. Set the pan aside for 5 minutes and allow it to cool.
10. Cut into square pieces and serve.

Veggie Coconut Chickpea Curry

Total Prep & Cooking Time: 50 minutes
Yields: Four Servings
Nutritional Facts: Calories: 300 | Protein: 17g | Fat: 8.2g | Carbs: 36g | Fiber: 16g

Ingredients:

- Two tsps. olive oil (extra virgin)
- One large red onion (chopped finely)
- Two tsps. fresh ginger (grated)
- Two cloves of garlic (crushed)
- Two tsps. mustard seeds (brown)
- One green chili (deseeded, chopped)
- Two tsps. curry powder
- 400 ml of vegetable stock
- 8 curry leaves (fresh)
- 150 ml coconut milk (reduced fat)
- 400 grams carrot (peeled, cubed)
- 300 grams of canned chickpeas (rinsed)
- 400 grams broccoli (cut into florets)
- One cup of peas (frozen)
- Two cups of quinoa (steamed, for serving)
- One cup of yogurt
- Fresh leaves of coriander (for serving)

Method:

1. Take a saucepan and add oil to it. Heat oil over a high flame and add onions to it.
2. Cook the onions for five minutes. Add ginger, garlic, curry leaves, and spices. Stir and cook for one more minute.
3. Add the milk and vegetable stock to the saucepan. Boil the mixture.
4. Add chickpeas along with carrots to the mixture. Reduce the flame and simmer the curry for 10 minutes. Stir the curry occasionally.

5. Add peas and broccoli to the mixture. Simmer it again for about 5 minutes or until the veggies are soft.
6. Serve the curry with yogurt, quinoa, and coriander from the top.

Zucchini Noodles With Cashews and Herbs

Total Prep & Cooking Time: 15 minutes
Yields: Four Servings
Nutritional Facts: Calories: 172 | Protein: 7g | Fat: 9g | Carbs: 13g |
Fiber: 8g

Ingredients:

- Four large-sized zucchinis (trimmed)
- Two corncobs (silk and husk removed)
- 300 grams cherry tomatoes (halved)
- One cup mint leaves (fresh)
- One-third cup of coriander leaves (fresh)
- One red chili (fresh, deseeded, chopped finely)
- Two tsps. tamari sauce
- One tbsp. lime juice
- One tsp. fresh ginger (grated)
- Half tsp. caster sugar
- Half cup unsalted cashews (roasted, chopped coarsely)

Method:

1. Start by cutting the zucchinis into noodle-like strands with the help of a spiralizer. In case you do not have a spiralizer, you can peel the zucchinis with the help of a vegetable peeler.
2. Cut the corn kernels by using a sharp knife.
3. Combine corn, zucchini, mint, tomato, along with coriander in a mixing bowl.
4. Add lime juice, chili, sugar, ginger, and tamari sauce in a bowl. Stir properly for dissolving the sugar.
5. Drizzle the prepared dressing over the zucchini noodle salad and toss for combining.
6. Serve in a plate with cashew from the top.

Lentil, Turmeric, and Lemon Soup

Total Prep & Cooking Time: 60 minutes
Yields: Four Servings
Nutritional Facts: Calories: 195 | Protein: 13g | Fat: 3.6g | Carbs: 26g | Fiber: 10.2g

Ingredients:

- One large onion (chopped finely)
- Two tsps. olive oil (extra virgin)
- Three stalks of celery (chopped finely)
- Two cloves of garlic (crushed)
- Two tsps. lemon rind (grated)
- One tsp. ground turmeric
- Half tsp. cinnamon (ground)
- Half tsp. chili flakes
- Two cups of vegetable stock
- Three-fourth cup of green lentils (rinsed)
- Two tomatoes (chopped)
- 200 grams green beans (sliced)
- 150 grams kale (chopped)
- One tbsp. lemon juice
- Two tbsps. fresh coriander (chopped)

Method:

1. Take a large saucepan and add olive oil to it—heat oil over a medium flame. Add celery and onions to the oil. Cook the onion for about five minutes or until tender. Add lemon rind, garlic, cinnamon, chili flakes, and turmeric to the pan. Cook the mixture for one minute and stir occasionally.
2. Add lentils, vegetable stock, three cups of water, and tomato to the saucepan. Boil the mixture.
3. Reduce the flame and cover the pan partially. Simmer the mixture for half an hour or until the lentils are soft.

4. Add kale and beans to the soup. Stir properly for combining. Simmer the soup for about four minutes or until the beans turn tender.
5. Add lemon juice to the soup and season by adding pepper.
6. Serve with coriander from the top.

Cabbage and Tamari Roasted Salad With Crunchy Noodle

Total Prep & Cooking Time: Twenty minutes
Yields: Four Servings
Nutritional Facts: Calories: 224 | Protein: 8.9g | Fat: 12.2g | Carbs: 19g | Fiber: 7.5g

Ingredients:
- Half cup mix of raw nibble (mix of almonds, sunflower seeds, raisins, pepitas, sultanas)
- Two tbsps. tamari sauce
- Three tbsps. lemon juice
- One tbsp. rice bran oil
- Half tbsp. sesame oil
- Two tsps. caster sugar
- One clove of garlic (crushed)
- One cm fresh ginger (grated)
- One red cabbage (shredded)
- One small broccoli (cut into florets)
- Four Brussels Sprouts (shredded)
- Two green onions (sliced thinly)
- 100 grams pack of fried noodles

Method:
1. Start by preheating the oven at 200 degrees Celsius. Use baking paper for lining a baking tray.
2. In a bowl, toss the nibble mix with tamari sauce. Spread the mix on the prepared tray. Roast the nibble mix for about 5 minutes. Stir the mix halfway.
3. Take a small bowl and add lime juice, sesame oil, sugar, rice bran oil, ginger, garlic, and the leftover tamari sauce. Whisk the mixture until the sugar gets dissolved.
4. In a large bowl, place broccoli, cabbage, onion, noodles, Brussels sprouts, and half of the nibble mix. Toss the ingredients for combining.
5. Add the dressing to the salad.
6. Sprinkle leftover nibble mix from the top. Serve with fried noodles.

Grilled Spicy Pumpkin With Tofu Salad

Total Prep & Cooking Time: 40 minutes
Yields: Four Servings
Nutritional Facts: Calories: 260 | Protein: 12g | Fat: 13g | Carbs: 19g | Fiber: 10g

Ingredients:

- One tbsp. honey
- One and a half tsps. cumin (ground)
- Two tsps. smoked paprika
- Half tsp. cinnamon (ground)
- Two tbsps. apple cider vinegar
- One tbsp. olive oil (extra virgin)
- 350 grams tofu (firm, sliced)
- 750 grams deseeded pumpkin (cut into wedges)
- One red deseeded capsicum (chopped)
- 250 grams of green beans (halved)
- Half cup parsley leaves (chopped)
- One tbsp. almond (chopped)

Method:

1. Mix one tsp. paprika, honey, one tsp. cumin, two tsps. vinegar, one-fourth tsp. cinnamon, and two tsps. oil in a bowl. Add tofu and pumpkin to the mix. Coat well.
2. Combine the leftover cumin, paprika, vinegar, cinnamon, and oil in another bowl and keep aside.
3. Preheat a chargrill or barbecue grill on medium. Add pumpkin to the grill. Cook both sides for about five minutes.
4. Cook the tofu on the grill for five minutes.
5. Spray the chopped capsicum with oil and cook until tender and charred.
6. Add the beans to a steamer and steam it for three minutes until tender.
7. Arrange pumpkin, tofu, beans, capsicum, and parsley on serving plates. Drizzle a bit of oil from the top.
8. Serve with chopped almonds from the top.

Chickpea Tagine

Total Prep & Cooking Time: 15 minutes
Yields: Four Servings
Nutritional Facts: Calories: 300 | Protein: 19g | Fat: 3.8g | Carbs: 52g | Fiber: 13g

Ingredients:

- Two 400 grams cans of chickpeas (rinsed)
- Two tbsps. Moroccan seasoning
- 400 grams canned tomatoes with garlic and onion (crushed)
- One cup couscous
- 70 grams baby spinach

Method:

1. Take a skillet and heat it over a medium flame. Add Moroccan seasoning along with chickpeas to the pan. Cook for two minutes, stirring occasionally.
2. Add half a cup of water and tomatoes to the pan. Boil the mixture.
3. Lower the flame. Simmer the mixture for about three minutes. Make sure the sauce thickens.
4. Place couscous in a bowl. Add one cup of boiling water to the bowl. Cover it with foil. Keep it aside for five minutes.
5. Separate the grains of couscous using a fork.
6. Serve the couscous with spinach and chickpea mixture.

Tofu Chili Zoodles

Total Prep & Cooking Time: Twenty minutes
Yields: Four Servings
Nutritional Facts: Calories: 190 | Protein: 10.2g | Fat: 13g | Carbs: 3g | Fiber: 8g

Ingredients:

- 400 grams of tofu (firm, cut into one cm cubes)
- Two tbsps. olive oil (chili-infused, extra virgin)
- Two large zucchini
- One large carrot (cut into matchsticks)
- One red chili (sliced)

Method:

1. Take the zucchini and make cut out strands with the use of a spiralizer. You can also use a vegetable peeler for peeling the zucchini.
2. Take a skillet and heat it over a medium flame. Add oil to the pan.
3. Add tofu to the skillet—Cook for five minutes. Keep the tofu aside.
4. Add zucchini to the pan and toss it for two minutes. Add carrots and toss for combining.
5. Add the cooked tofu to the zucchini mixture and toss again for combining.
6. Serve with chili and remaining oil from the top.

Spicy Moroccan Tomato and Eggplant

Total Prep & Cooking Time: 40 minutes
Yields: Four Servings
Nutritional Facts: Calories: 113 | Protein: 4g | Fat: 3.5g | Carbs: 11g
| Fiber: 5.2g

Ingredients:

- Three eggplants (trimmed)
- Five medium-sized tomatoes
- Twp tsps. olive oil (extra virgin)
- Two cloves of garlic (crushed)
- One tbsp. harissa paste
- 300 grams cherry tomatoes
- Two tbsps. parsley leaves (chopped finely)
- Two tbsps. mint leaves (fresh, chopped)
- Lemon wedges (for serving)

Method:

1. Place the eggplants in a bowl. Cover the bowl with the help of plastic wrap. Microwave, the eggplants on a high setting for five minutes or until the eggplants are tender. Keep the eggplants aside for cooling. Cut the eggplants in halves and chop them roughly.
2. Use a small knife and remove the cores from the tomatoes.
3. Place the tomatoes in a bowl and add boiling water to it.
4. Keep the tomatoes in boiling water for sixty seconds. Drain the tomato water and wash the tomatoes under running cold water. Peel the tomato skin and roughly chop the tomatoes.
5. Take a pan and heat it over a medium flame. Add oil to the pan.
6. Add harissa and garlic to the oil—Cook for about one minute. Add the chopped tomatoes to the pan and simmer.
7. Simmer the tomato mixture for about ten minutes and add the cherry tomatoes. Cook for five minutes or until the tomato turns soft.

8. Add parsley, eggplant, and mint to the tomato mix—season with pepper and salt.
9. Toss the mixture for one minute.
10. Serve with wedges of lemon by the side.

Lemon Broccoli Soup With Feta and Quinoa

Total Prep & Cooking Time: 30 minutes
Yields: Four Servings
Nutritional Facts: Calories: 268 | Protein: 15g | Fat: 11.9g | Carbs: 20g | Fiber: 7.5g

Ingredients:

- One-third cup quinoa (tri-colored)
- One cup of water
- One tbsp. olive oil (extra-virgin)
- One large onion (chopped)
- Two cloves of garlic (crushed)
- Two large potatoes (peeled and chopped)
- One large broccoli (separate the florets and stems)
- Four cups vegetable stock
- 100 grams spinach (baby leaves)
- Half cup mint leaves
- Two tbsps. lemon juice
- Two tsps. lemon rind (grated)
- 30 grams feta (crumbled)
- Baby herbs (for serving)

Method:

1. Take a saucepan and add quinoa along with 150 ml water. Bring the mixture to boil—Cook for twelve minutes. Make sure the quinoa is tender. Drain the water and wash it under cold water.
2. Take a saucepan and heat it over medium flame. Add oil to the pan. Add garlic and onion to the pan—Cook the mixture for four to five minutes.
3. Add the broccoli stems and potato to the pan. Add water along with the stock. Boil the mixture.
4. Lower the flame. Simmer for about ten minutes. Make sure that the potatoes are soft.

5. Add the florets of broccoli to the mixture. Simmer for another five minutes.
6. Add mint and spinach to the mixture. Simmer for two minutes until the spinach wilts.
7. Use a hand blender for processing the soup until smooth.
8. Add lemon juice and give the soup a stir.
9. Divide the soup among bowls and top with lemon rind, quinoa, baby herbs, and feta. You can also drizzle some olive oil from the top.

Mixed Veggie Curry

Total Prep & Cooking Time: 60 minutes
Yields: Four Servings
Nutritional Facts: Calories: 170 | Protein: 6g | Fat: 3.8g | Carbs: 24g | Fiber: 8.5g

Ingredients:
- One tbsp. vegetable oil
- One large onion (sliced thinly)
- Three carrots (sliced)
- Three large potatoes (cut into 3 cm pieces)
- Half cauliflower (cut into florets)
- One medium eggplant (sliced)
- One-fourth tsp. ground turmeric
- Two tsps. fennel seeds
- Three cloves of garlic (chopped)
- One tsp. chili powder
- 2 cm fresh ginger (chopped)
- 400 grams of canned tomatoes
- One stick of cinnamon
- Four curry leaves (fresh)
- Coriander leaves (fresh, for serving)

Method:
1. Take a saucepan and heat it over medium flame. Add oil to the pan. Add onion to the pan. Sauté for about ten minutes.
2. Add potato and carrot to the onion—Cook for five minutes. Stir occasionally.
3. Add eggplant and cauliflower to the mixture and cook for one minute.
4. Add turmeric, chili, fennels seeds, ginger, and garlic. Cook for two more minutes and stir continuously.
5. Add curry leaves, tomato, one cup of water, and cinnamon to the pan. Bring the mixture to simmer.
6. Reduce the flame and simmer for twenty minutes.
7. Check if the vegetables are tender. If needed, simmer the curry for some more time.
8. Serve with coriander from the top.

Peach Panzanella

Total Prep & Cooking Time: Twenty minutes
Yields: Four Servings
Nutritional Facts: Calories: 322 | Protein: 15g | Fat: 21g | Carbs: 32g | Fiber: 7.5g

Ingredients:

- Two tbsps. balsamic vinegar (white)
- One tbsp. lemon juice
- Half tsp. Dijon mustard
- 80 ml of olive oil (extra virgin)
- 400 grams baby tomatoes (halved)
- Two large tomatoes (halved)
- One red capsicum (deseeded, chopped)
- One red onion (sliced)
- Three peaches (quartered)
- 200 grams of ciabatta bread
- 120 grams of goat's cheese (crumbled)
- One clove of garlic (halved)
- Two cups fresh herbs (firmly packed)

Method:

1. Mix lemon juice, vinegar, two tbsps. of oil, and mustard in a jar. Season with pepper and salt. Shake well for combining.
2. Take a bowl and combine onion, tomatoes, and capsicum. Add half of the prepared dressing. Toss properly for coating. Keep it aside for developing the flavors.
3. Preheat a chargrill or barbecue grill on medium.
4. Mix two tsps. of oil and peach in a mixing bowl. Season pepper and salt.
5. Cook the pepper in the grill for about four minutes or until tender and charred. Transfer the grilled peaches to a plate.
6. Use the remaining oil for brushing the bread.
7. Add bread to the grill—Cook for five minutes or until charred.

8. Remove the bread from the grill and rub it with the cut side of the clove of garlic. Tear the bread coarsely.
9. Add herbs, cheese, bread, and peach to the mixture of tomatoes.
10. Add the remaining dressing and toss gently for combining.
11. Serve immediately.

Buckwheat Pasta With Chickpeas and Roast Cauliflower

Total Prep & Cooking Time: 40 minutes
Yields: Four Servings
Nutritional Facts: Calories: 321 | Protein: 14g | Fat: 6g | Carbs: 41g | Fiber: 13g

Ingredients:

- One small cauliflower
- Two tsps. balsamic vinegar
- Two tbsps. currants
- 250 grams buckwheat pasta
- One tbsp. olive oil
- Four shallots (sliced)
- Two cloves of garlic (crushed)
- Two tsps. lemon rind
- 400 grams of canned chickpeas
- One-third cup vegetable stock
- 100 grams spinach (baby)
- Half cup parsley (fresh)
- One tbsp. lemon juice (fresh)

Method:

1. Preheat the oven at a temperature of 180 degrees Celsius. Use baking paper for lining a baking sheet. Place florets of cauliflower on the sheet and spray with oil—Bake for half an hour.
2. Cook the pasta in a pan with salted water. Drain the pasta.
3. Heat two tsps. of oil in an iron skillet over a medium flame. Add garlic, shallot, and lemon rind. Add vinegar and currants—Cook for two minutes.
4. Add the stock and chickpeas to the pan.
5. Add spinach to the pan and cook until it wilts.
6. Add the cauliflower, chickpea mixture, lemon juice, parsley, and two tsps. oil to the cooked pasta. Toss properly.
7. Season and serve with parsley from the top.

Cashew-Cauliflower Soup and Crispy Buckwheat

Total Prep & Cooking Time: 40 minutes
Yields: 2 Serving
Nutrition Facts: Calories: 240 | Protein: 7g | Fat: 19g | Carbs: 17g |
Fiber: 5g

Ingredients:

- Half cup olive oil (extra virgin)
- Four shallots (sliced)
- Two cloves of garlic (sliced)
- One bay leaf
- One cup white wine (dry)
- Kosher salt
- One cauliflower (cut in florets, chopped stem)
- One-fourth tsp. cayenne pepper
- Three tbsps. cashew
- Seven cups of vegetable stock
- Two tsps. pepper (ground)
- Two tbsps. of buckwheat groats
- Three tsps. lemon juice
- Half tsp. paprika

Method:

1. Take a pot and heat it over medium flame—heat one-fourth cup of oil in the pot. Add bay leaf, garlic, shallots, and thyme—Cook for eight minutes. Stir occasionally.
2. Add white wine to the pot. Boil the mixture. Keep cooking until the mixture gets reduced by half. Add three-fourth cup cauliflower to the pot and three-fourth cup cashews to the pot. Add cayenne and give it a stir.
3. Cover the pot and cook until the cauliflower is tender.
4. Add vegetable stock to the pot and add salt along with pepper. Bring the soup to boil. Simmer for half an hour. Remove bay leaf from the soup.
5. Chop the remaining cauliflower and cashews.

6. Heat oil in a skillet over a medium flame. Add cashews, cauliflower, and groats. Add salt according to taste. Cook until the ingredients are brown in color. Remove the pan from the heat and add paprika along with lemon juice.
7. Puree the prepared soup using a hand blender until creamy and smooth. Reheat the soup over a low flame, and you can add more vegetable stock if required.
8. Serve the soup in bowls with buckwheat-cauliflower mixture from the top.

CHAPTER 4:
RECIPES FOR POULTRY

Chicken and eggs can act as great companions for your weight-loss regime, especially for Sirtfood Diet. So, I have included some tasty poultry recipes in this chapter for giving a good dose of protein to your daily diet plan.

Creamy Pea and Chicken Pasta

Total Prep & Cooking Time: 25 minutes
Yields: Four Servings
Nutritional Facts: Calories: 323 | Protein: 35g | Fat: 9.5g | Carbs: 28g | Fiber: 12g

Ingredients:

- 200 grams of chickpea pasta
- Three-fourth cup of peas (frozen)
- 150 grams of peas (sugar snap, halved)
- Two tsps. olive oil (extra virgin)
- 300 grams of chicken breast
- Twelve cherry tomatoes
- Three cloves of garlic (crushed)
- Half tsp. chili flakes
- Two tsps lemon rind (grated)
- One large egg
- One-fourth cup cream (light)
- Three tbsps. lemon juice (fresh)
- 20 grams parmesan (grated)
- 80 grams rocket arugula

Method:

1. Take a saucepan and start cooking the pasta in boiling water. Add some salt to the water.

2. Cook the pasta until al dente and add sugar snap peas along with frozen pas for the last one minute of cooking.
3. Keep aside one-fourth cup of the pasta liquid.
4. Drain the pasta and keep it aside.
5. Take a skillet and heat it over a medium flame. Add oil to the pan. Add tomatoes and chicken to the skillet. Cook the mixture for four to five minutes or until the chicken is cooked properly.
6. Add chili flakes, garlic, and lemon rind to the pan. Cook for one minute or until you can smell the aroma.
7. Whisk together cream, egg, parmesan, and lemon juice in a mixing bowl.
8. Add the mixture of egg and along with the chicken to the pasta. Toss the pasta for coating in the sauce. Add some of the pasta liquid and cook for sixty seconds.
9. Add arugula to the pasta and toss again.
10. Serve the pasta with parmesan from the top.

Stir Fry Chicken Satay

Total Prep & Cooking Time: Twenty minutes
Yields: Four Servings
Nutritional Facts: Calories: 360 | Protein: 30g | Fat: 12g | Carbs: 36g | Fiber: 7.9g

Ingredients:

- One-fourth cup coconut milk (light)
- Two tbsps. peanut butter (crunchy)
- Two tsps. olive oil
- 500 grams of chicken tenderloins
- Two cloves of garlic (chopped)
- Two tsps. ginger (chopped)
- 400 grams pumpkin (peeled, deseeded, chopped)
- One bunch of broccolini (halved)
- Red chili (optional)
- Coriander sprigs (for serving)
- Steamed rice (for serving)
- Halves of lime (for serving)

Method:

1. Combine peanut butter and coconut milk in a bowl. Keep it aside for later usage.
2. Take a wok and heat it over a high flame. Add oil to the wok. Add the chicken tenderloins to the oil and cook for about three minutes. Transfer the chicken to a bowl and let it cool. Chop the chicken into thirds.
3. Add ginger and garlic to the wok. Stir fry the mixture for one minute or until you can smell the aroma. Add pumpkin to the wok and cook week for coating. Add one-third cup of water to the wok and cook for five minutes.
4. Add broccolini to the wok and cover—Cook for three more minutes or until soft.
5. Add coconut milk mixture and chicken to the wok.
6. Toss properly for coating.
7. Simmer the mixture for two minutes for making the sauce thick.
8. Serve with rice and lime halves. Garnish with coriander and chili from the top.

Coconut and Chicken Curry

Total Prep & Cooking Time: 40 minutes
Yields: Four Servings
Nutritional Facts: Calories: 350 | Protein: 38g | Fat: 12g | Carbs: 28g | Fiber: 8g

Ingredients:
- One red onion
- Two cloves of garlic (chopped)
- Two tsps. fresh ginger (grated)
- Three red chilis (chopped)
- One stick of lemongrass (chopped)
- Half cup chopped stems of coriander
- One lime (half zest, half juiced)
- Three tsps. macadamia oil
- 600 grams of chicken breast (chopped)
- One cup of coconut milk (light)
- Half cup chicken stock
- 400 grams pumpkin (cut into cubes)
- 200 grams of green beans (halved)
- 200 grams of snow peas (diagonally halved)
- One tsp. fish sauce
- Two cups of quinoa (cooked)

Method:
1. Chop half of the onion. Slice the other half. Take a food processor and process garlic, chopped onion, lemongrass, chili, ginger, lime zest, coriander, and two tsps. of oil. Make a paste.
2. Take a saucepan and heat oil in it over a medium flame. Add sliced onion to it along with the curry paste—Cook for five minutes.
3. Add chicken and cook until browned. Add stock, pumpkin, and coconut milk. Bring the mixture to a boil.
4. Add beans to the pan and simmer for ten minutes. Add fish sauce along with lime juice.
5. Serve with cooked quinoa with coriander from the top.

One Pan Chicken

Total Prep & Cooking Time: 15 minutes
Yields: Four Servings
Nutritional Facts: Calories: 368 | Protein: 50g | Fat: 17g | Carbs: 16g | Fiber: 3.6g

Ingredients:

- Half shallot (chopped)
- One clove of garlic (chopped)
- Two tbsps. olive oil (extra virgin)
- Half cup basil leaves (chopped)
- Two breasts of chicken (halved)
- 250 grams baby tomatoes (halved)
- Four bocconcini (sliced)
- One tbsp. red wine vinegar
- One tsp. caster sugar
- Crusty bread (for serving)

Method:

1. Take a bowl and mix garlic, shallot, basil, and one tbsp. oil. Season the mixture.
2. Heat a pan and add oil to it. Season the pieces of chicken and add to the pan—Cook for five minutes. Make sure the chicken is golden in color.
3. Preheat your oven to high.
4. Add tomato to the chicken along with half of the basil mixture.
5. Sprinkle vinegar from the top.
6. Top the chicken with bocconcini.
7. Grill for about five minutes or until the cheese gets melted.
8. Serve with basil from the top along with bread.

Healthy Chicken Korma

Total Prep & Cooking Time: 45 minutes
Yields: Four Servings
Nutritional Facts: Calories: 320 | Protein: 32g | Fat: 11.2g | Carbs: 23g | Fiber: 10g

Ingredients:

- Two tsps. macadamia oil
- 500 grams of chicken breast (sliced)
- Two onions (sliced)
- Two tbsps. korma paste
- One stick of cinnamon
- Eight pods of cardamom (crushed)
- Half tsp. chicken stock powder
- Two carrots (sliced)
- 200 grams of green beans (halved)
- One bunch broccolini
- One-fourth cup plain yogurt
- One tbsp. almond meal

Method:

1. Take a skillet and add oil to it—heat oil over a medium flame.
2. Add chicken to the oil and cook for three minutes.
3. Heat the remaining oil in another pan over a high flame. Add the onions and cook them for four minutes. Add korma paste, pods of cardamom, and cinnamon stick.
4. Cook for two minutes and stir occasionally.
5. Add one cup of water to the pan along with the stock powder. Add the carrots.
6. Add chicken to the pan. Boil the mixture.
7. Cover the pan and reduce the flame. Simmer for about ten minutes or until the carrots are soft.
8. Add broccolini and beans to the pan. Simmer for five more minutes or until all the veggies are soft. Remove the stick of cinnamon.
9. Remove the pan from heat and add yogurt to the korma.
10. Serve hot with roti.

Cumin Chicken With Chickpea Salsa

Total Prep & Cooking Time: 45 minutes
Yields: Four Servings
Nutritional Facts: Calories: 350 | Protein: 42g | Fat: 8g | Carbs: 25g
| Fiber: 10g

Ingredients:

- Two tsps. cumin (ground)
- Half tsp. chili flakes
- Two fillets of chicken breast (halved)
- One tbsp. olive oil
- 800 grams pumpkin (cut in wedges)
- Two tbsps. lemon juice
- One small onion (chopped)
- Two cloves of garlic (crushed)
- Two tbsps. currants
- 350 grams of canned chickpeas (rinsed)
- Half cup coriander (chopped)
- One tbsp. lemon zest

Method:

1. Mix chili flakes and cumin in a small bowl. Sprinkle half of the mixture over chicken pieces with one tsp. oil.
2. Cook the pumpkin in a microwave-safe bowl for five minutes or until soft. Season with oil and salt.
3. Heat a chargrill or barbecue grill over a medium flame—Cook the microwaved pumpkin for four minutes.
4. Add chicken to grill—Cook the chicken for six minutes. Make sure the chicken is tender. Add one tsp. of lemon juice from the top.
5. Take a pan and heat oil in it over a medium flame. Add garlic, onion, spice mix, and currants to the oil and cook for five minutes. Add the chickpeas and cook for two more minutes.
6. Add lemon zest, lemon juice, and coriander to the pan.
7. Serve the chicken and pumpkin with chickpea salsa.

Caper and Lemon Grilled Chicken With Caprese Salad

Total Prep & Cooking Time: 55 minutes
Yields: Four Servings
Nutritional Facts: Calories: 250 | Protein: 26g | Fat: 12g | Carbs: 3.1g | Fiber: 6g

Ingredients:

- Two tbsps. lemon juice
- One tbsp. vinegar (balsamic)
- One tbsp. olive oil
- One tsp. lemon rind
- One tbsp. baby capers (rinsed, chopped)
- Four fillets of chicken breast
- Two bunches of asparagus (trimmed)
- 300 grams of tomato medley (halved)
- Half cup basil leaves
- 70 grams arugula
- 60 grams bocconcini
- One tbsp. sunflower seeds (toasted)

Method:

1. Mix vinegar, lemon juice, olive oil, capers, and lemon rind in a small bowl.
2. Take a shallow dish and marinate the chicken pieces with half of the dressing. Marinate for twenty minutes.
3. Preheat a chargrill or barbecue grill. Spray the asparagus and chicken with oil—Cook the chicken for five minutes and the asparagus for two minutes.
4. Slice the cooked chicken and keep it aside.
5. Cut grilled asparagus in half. Mix tomato, asparagus, basil, arugula, and bocconcini in a mixing bowl. Add the remaining dressing and toss.
6. Serve in plates and top with cooked chicken.
7. Sprinkle sunflower seeds from the top.

Sweet Potatoes With Jalapeno Slaw and Chicken

Total Prep & Cooking Time: One hour and twenty-five minutes
Yields: Four Servings
Nutritional Facts: Calories: 345 | Protein: 22g | Fat: 4g | Carbs: 27g
| Fiber: 15g

Ingredients:

- Four small sweet potatoes
- 500 grams canned black beans (rinsed)
- 150 grams cooked chicken (chopped)
- One ripe tomato (diced)
- Three shallots (sliced)
- One green chili (deseeded, chopped)
- One cup cottage cheese
- Two tbsps. coriander (chopped)
- Two cups red cabbage (chopped)
- Two tsps. lime juice
- One tsp. olive oil

Method:

1. Preheat oven at 180 degrees Celsius. Use baking paper for lining a baking sheet.
2. Take the sweet potatoes and prick them all over with a fork. Place the potatoes on the tray and bake for about one hour or until soft.
3. Mix chicken, tomato, black beans, chili, shallot, cottage cheese, and half coriander in a bowl.
4. Combine jalapeno, cabbage, coriander, olive oil, and lemon juice in another bowl.
5. Remove the potato skin and mash them with a fork. Bake for another five minutes.
6. Serve with jalapeno slaw and chicken mix.

Lemon Chicken and Noodle Salad

Total Prep & Cooking Time: 60 minutes
Yields: Four Servings
Nutritional Facts: Calories: 285 | Protein: 33g | Fat: 3.9g | Carbs: 23g | Fiber: 8g

Ingredients:

- 500 grams fillets of chicken breast
- One stem of lemongrass (chopped)
- One tsp. lemon rind (grated)
- Half tsp. turmeric
- Two red chilies (chopped, deseeded)
- One-third cup lemon juice
- 100 grams of egg noodles
- One red onion (sliced)
- 100 grams of snap peas (sliced)
- One red cabbage (shredded)
- 100 grams grape tomatoes (halved)
- One cup mint leaves
- Half cup coriander leaves (chopped)
- Two tsps. fish sauce
- One and a half tsps. brown sugar

Method:

1. Mix lemongrass, chicken, turmeric, lemon rind, half chili, and two tbsps. of lemon juice in a bowl. Place the mix in the freezer for half an hour.
2. Cook the egg noodles and drain. Wash under cold water.
3. Take a large work and heat it over a high flame. Add oil to the wok and cook the chicken for four minutes or until browned.
4. Add onion, noodles, peas, tomato, cabbage, mint, and coriander to the cooked chicken.
5. Mix sugar, fish sauce, chili, and lemon juice in a bowl.
6. Add the prepared dressing to the chicken salad. Toss for combining.

Baked Eggs and Tapenade Toast

Total Prep & Cooking Time: 35 minutes
Yields: Four Servings
Nutritional Facts: Calories: 312 | Protein: 19g | Fat: 13g | Carbs: 27g
| Fiber: 10.2g

Ingredients:

- Two tbsps. olive oil (extra virgin)
- Two red capsicums (sliced)
- One yellow capsicum (sliced)
- One red onion (sliced)
- Two cloves of garlic (crushed)
- Three tomatoes (chopped)
- Two tsps. red wine vinegar
- One-fourth tsp. brown sugar
- One-third cup basil (torn)
- Four large eggs
- Eight slices of toasted baguette

Method:

1. Take a skillet and heat oil in it over a medium flame. Add the capsicums to the oil—Cook for two minutes. Add garlic and onion. Season with pepper along with salt. Cook for ten minutes.
2. Add tomato to mixture pan and cook for five minutes. Add sugar, vinegar, and basil.
3. Use a spoon for making four wells in the mixture of capsicum. Crack one egg in each well. Reduce the flame.
4. Cover the pan. Cook for ten minutes. Make sure the yolk gets cooked.
5. Serve with baguette toasts and basil from the top.

Green Pasta With Creamy Chicken

Total Prep & Cooking Time: 25 minutes
Yields: Four Servings
Nutritional Facts: Calories: 360 | Protein: 25g | Fat: 11g | Carbs: 39g | Fiber: 8.3g

Ingredients:

- 400 grams spelt pasta
- One bunch broccolini
- One bunch asparagus (cut into 3 cm length)
- Three shallots (sliced)
- Two cloves of garlic (crushed)
- Two zucchini (shredded)
- 250 grams of light cream
- Half cup chicken stock
- 250 grams of barbecued chicken (shredded)
- Half cup parsley (for serving)

Method:

1. Cook pasta in a saucepan with boiling water. Add asparagus and broccolini to the pan for the last minutes of cooking. Drain the ingredients.
2. Take a skillet and heat it over a medium flame. Add oil to the pan. Cook the sliced shallots in the pan for one minute and add garlic to it. Cook for about thirty seconds and add zucchini to the pan. Cook the mixture for one minute.
3. Add stock and cream to the pan. Simmer the mixture for two minutes.
4. Add chicken to the sauce and stir well for combining.
5. Add pasta to the chicken mixture and toss.
6. Season with salt and pepper. Serve with parsley from the top.

Watercress Salad With Asparagus and Chicken

Total Prep & Cooking Time: 60 minutes
Yields: Four Servings
Nutritional Facts: Calories: 350 | Protein: 42g | Fat: 11g | Carbs: 27g | Fiber: 10.3g

Ingredients:

- 600 grams of chicken breast
- Two cloves of garlic (crushed)
- Two tbsps. lemon juice
- One tbsp. olive oil
- Two bunches of asparagus (halved)
- 200 grams of snow peas (trimmed)
- Half bunch watercress
- 400 grams canned brown lentils (rinsed)

For Dressing:

- One tbsp. of lemon juice
- One tsp. of lemon zest
- One tbsp. of orange juice
- Two tsps. of poppy seeds
- Twp tsp. honey
- Half cup sour cream

Method:
1. Cut the breasts of chicken into thin slices.
2. Add lemon juice, garlic, and oil in a shallow dish. Add the chicken pieces and coat. Marinate for half an hour.
3. Heat a grill pan over a high flame. Cook the chicken for three minutes or until charred.
4. Blanch the asparagus along with peas in a saucepan with boiling water. Wash under cold water. Drain the water.
5. Take a bowl and mix snow peas, lentils, and watercress.
6. Combine all the ingredients for the dressing.
7. Serve the asparagus and chicken with dressing from the top.

Stir-Fry Hoisin Chicken

Total Prep & Cooking Time: 45 minutes
Yields: Four Servings
Nutritional Facts: Calories: 308 | Protein: 26g | Fat: 20g | Carbs: 12g | Fiber: 9g

Ingredients:

- 400 grams chicken breast (sliced)
- Half cup hoisin sauce
- 80 ml of peanut oil
- Two cloves of garlic (sliced)
- Three cm ginger (julienne)
- One red onion (cut in wedges)
- One bunch pay choy (chopped)
- One red capsicum(sliced)
- One yellow capsicum (sliced)
- Two spring onions (sliced)

Method:

1. Take a bowl and combine chicken with two tbsps. of hoisin sauce. Season the chicken with pepper and salt. Marinate for 20 minutes.
2. Heat two tbsps. of olive oil in a wok and add chicken to it. Stir-fry the chicken for five minutes or until browned. Transfer chicken to a bowl.
3. Add two tbsps. oil to the wok. Add ginger, garlic, beans, red onion, pak choy, and capsicums to the wok. Fry for two minutes. Add chicken to the wok along with the remaining hoisin sauce. Add two tbsps. of water.
4. Stir-fry the chicken mix for three minutes.
5. Serve with rice.

Healthy Veggie and Chicken Stir-Fry

Total Prep & Cooking Time: 35 minutes
Yields: Four Servings
Nutritional Facts: Calories: 308 | Protein: 33g | Fat: 5g | Carbs: 28g
| Fiber: 8g

Ingredients:

- 100 grams vermicelli noodles
- Two tbsps. tamari
- One tbsp. lime juice
- One tsp. brown sugar
- 500 grams of chicken breast (sliced)
- One red onion (sliced)
- One carrot (sliced)
- One red chili (chopped)
- One stalk of lemongrass (chopped)
- Two tsps. fresh ginger (grated)
- Two cloves of garlic (chopped)
- One red capsicum (sliced)
- 200 grams snap peas (trimmed)
- 250 grams zucchini noodles
- Basil leaves (for serving)

Method:
1. Soak the noodles in boiling water for five minutes. Drain the noodles and keep aside.
2. Combine lime juice, tamari, and sugar in a bowl. Keep stirring until the sugar dissolves.
3. Take a wok and heat oil in it. Add carrot and onion to the wok and stir-fry for two minutes. Add lemongrass, chili, garlic along with ginger—Cook for sixty seconds. Add peas, capsicum, and two tbsps. water to the wok. Stir-fry for one minute. Add vermicelli noodles and zucchini to the mixture and stir-fry for three minutes.
4. Add chicken and sauce mix and cook for about two minutes.
5. Serve with basil from the top.

Sweet Potato Bowl and Mexican Beans

Total Prep & Cooking Time: 40 minutes
Yields: Four Servings
Nutritional Facts: Calories: 300 | Protein: 13g | Fat: 11g | Carbs: 26g | Fiber: 10g

Ingredients:

- 500 grams sweet potato (cut in 2 cm pieces)
- One tsp. olive oil
- One red onion (chopped)
- Two cloves of garlic (crushed)
- One tsp. paprika
- One tsp. cumin (ground)
- Two large tomatoes (chopped)
- 400 grams canned black beans (rinsed)
- Four eggs
- 100 grams arugula
- Half avocado (mashed)
- Two tsps. chili sauce

Method:

1. Preheat oven at 180 degrees Celsius. Use baking paper for lining a baking sheet. Add potato to the tray and spray with oil—Bake for half an hour or until soft.
2. Heat the oil in a pan. Add onion to the oil—Cook for six minutes. Add paprika and garlic. Stir for one minute. Add black beans, cumin, and tomato to the mixture—Cook for five minutes. Mash the beans using a fork.
3. Take another pan and heat oil in it. Fry eggs in the oil and remove from the pan.
4. Divide the sweet potato, arugula, and bean mixture among four bowls. Top each bowl with fried egg and avocado. Drizzle chili sauce from the top and serve.

Cajun Charred Chicken With Broccoli Salad

Total Prep & Cooking Time: 35 minutes
Yields: Four Servings
Nutritional Facts: Calories: 360 | Protein: 40g | Fat: 25g | Carbs: 5g | Fiber: 9.3g

Ingredients:

- Four chicken thighs
- Two tbsps. Cajun seasoning
- One-fourth cup olive oil (extra virgin)
- 300 grams broccoli (cut into florets)
- One carrot (grated)
- One red onion (sliced)
- Half cup lemon juice
- One tbsp. baby capers (drained)
- One lemon (cut in wedges, for serving)

Method:

1. Score the chicken thighs for three times. Place the chicken thighs on a plate and season. Add some oil to the chicken and coat.
2. Heat a grill pan—Cook the chicken for twenty minutes. Make sure the chicken is properly cooked.
3. Chop the florets of broccoli into small pieces. Grate the stems of broccoli. Add onion, carrot, capers, lemon juice, and oil. Season with pepper and salt. Toss for combining.
4. Serve the chicken with lemon wedges and salad.

Feta Omelet and Broccoli With Toast

Total Prep & Cooking Time: 15 minutes
Yields: 1 Serving
Nutrition Facts: Calories: 330 | Protein: 24g | Fat: 14g | Carbs: 31g
| Fiber: 8g

Ingredients:

- Cooking Spray
- Two large eggs
- One cup broccoli florets (chopped)
- Twp tbsps. feta cheese (crumbled)
- One-fourth tsp. dried dill
- Two slices bread (toasted)

Method:

1. Heat a skillet and spray cooking oil. Add chopped broccoli to the oil and cook for four minutes.
2. Mix feta, eggs, and dill in a bowl. Add the egg mixture to the pan and cook for five minutes. Turn the omelet and keep cooking for another minute.
3. Serve hot with toast.

Chicken Mole Enchiladas

Total Prep & Cooking Time: 50 minutes
Yields: Four Servings
Nutritional Facts: Calories: 240 | Protein: 13g | Fat:7.9g | Carbs: 27g | Fiber: 5.4g

Ingredients:

- Two cups of chicken broth
- Eight ounces of mole negro sauce
- Four cups of cooked chicken (shredded)
- Eight tortillas (corn)
- Half cup feta (crumbled)
- Half red onion (sliced in rings)

Method:

1. Take a saucepan and mix chicken broth and negro sauce. Simmer the dressing for fifteen minutes. You can use more chicken broth if needed.
2. Heat the cooked chicken in a microwave for one minute.
3. Take a mixing bowl and add chicken and mole. Toss properly for coating the chicken with a layer of mole sauce.
4. Heat a skillet over medium flame.
5. When the skillet gets hot, add the tortillas and toast on both sides.
6. Add a scoop of tossed chicken in each tortilla. Roll in the shape of a burrito.
7. Serve with mole sauce from the top.

Baked Eggs and Beans

Total Prep & Cooking Time: 25 minutes
Yields: 2 Servings
Nutrition Facts: Calories: 180 | Protein: 10g | Fat:2.9g | Carbs: 13g
| Fiber: 3.7g

Ingredients:

- One onion (sliced)
- Two tomatoes (sliced)
- Two tbsps. of olive oil
- One lemon
- Half tbsp. of cumin (ground)
- One tsp. red chili (dry)
- 300 grams of boiled beans
- Two tbsps. of tomato sauce
- Four eggs
- Spring onions
- One tbsp. honey
  Three tbsps. cheese (grated)
- Half cup coriander (chopped)

Method:

1. Start by preheating your oven at 180 degrees Celsius.
2. Take a pan and heat it over medium flame. Add olive oil to the pan. Add some red chilies and cumin.
3. Add the sliced tomatoes and onions to the pan.
4. Add salt, beans, pepper, lemon juice, and coriander to the pan—Cook for five minutes.
5. Add the honey and tomato sauce to the pan.
6. Break the eggs in the prepared mixture. Put the mixture in the preheated oven for about ten minutes. Make sure the eggs get cooked properly.
7. Serve with coriander and onions from the top.

CHAPTER 5:
RECIPES FOR SEAFOOD

There are various seafood items that can be included in your Sirtfood Diet plan. In this chapter, you will find some tasty seafood recipes that you can include in your Sirtfood Diet.

Prawn Tacos and Bean Salad

Total Prep & Cooking Time: 60 minutes
Yields: Four Servings
Nutritional Facts: Calories: 329 | Protein: 36g | Fat: 7.6g | Carbs: 29.3g | Fiber: 13g

Ingredients:

- One-third cup coriander leaves (packed firmly)
- One red chili (chopped)
- Two tsps. paprika
- One and a half tbsps. lime juice
- One tbsp. olive oil
- 500 grams prawns (peeled)
- One red onion (chopped)
- Two cloves of garlic (crushed)
- 400 grams canned black beans (rinsed)
- Two tomatoes
- 200 grams green beans (sliced)
- Eight tortillas (corn, chargrilled)
- Half cup yogurt (Greek)
- Lime wedges (for serving)
- Coriander leaves (for serving)

Method:

1. Process chili, coriander, and half of the paprika in a blender. Add two tsps. oil and lime juice and process again. You can also add some water to make the paste smooth.
2. Marinate the prawns with the paste and keep it aside for half an hour.
3. Take an iron skillet and heat oil in it over a medium flame. Add onion to the pan and cook for five minutes. Add paprika and garlic to the pan along with the black beans. Give it a stir and add the tomatoes. Simmer for three minutes.
4. Heat a grill pan over a high flame. Cook the marinated prawns for two minutes on both sides.
5. Top the tortillas with bean salad, a dollop of yogurt, and cooked prawns.
6. Serve with wedges of lime and coriander from the top.

Salmon, Broccoli, and Chia Fish Cakes

Total Prep & Cooking Time: 60 minutes
Yields: Four Servings
Nutritional Facts: Calories: 317 | Protein: 28g | Fat: 12.3g | Carbs: 20g | Fiber: 11.2g

Ingredients:

- 400 grams sweet potato (peeled, cut into pieces of 3 cm)
- 250 grams broccoli florets
- 400 grams canned pink or red salmon (flaked, drained)
- Four green shallots (chopped)
- Half cup quinoa flakes
- Two tbsps. chia seeds
- Three tbsps. parsley (chopped)
- Two tbsps. fresh dill (chopped)
- Two tsps. lemon rind (grated)
- Low-fat yogurt (for serving)
- Mixed leaves of salad (for serving)
- Wedges of baby cucumber (for serving)

Method:

1. Start by steaming the potatoes for ten minutes or until soft. Mash the potatoes using a fork and allow it to cool.
2. Steam or boil the broccoli florets for two minutes or until tender. Drain the water and chop finely.
3. Add the broccoli to the sweet potato along with the salmon, quinoa flakes, green shallot, chia, dill, lemon rind, and parsley. Season properly and mix well.
4. Divide the mixture into eight portions. Wet your hands and shape each portion into a thick patty of two cm. Keep the patty on a large plate.
5. Place the patty in the freezer for half an hour.
6. Take a frying pan and spray oil in it. Heat it over medium flame. Start cooking the fish cakes for three minutes on each side until browned.
7. Serve with salad leaves, cucumber, and yogurt.

Crispy Lettuce and Salmon With Pearl Couscous

Total Prep & Cooking Time: Twenty minutes
Yields: Four Servings
Nutritional Facts: Calories: 304 | Protein: 26g | Fat: 12g | Carbs: 32g | Fiber: 7.2g

Ingredients:

- 150 grams pearl couscous
- 160 grams baby kale
- Two zucchini (shredded)
- Two shallots (chopped)
- 100 grams pea sprouts
- 300 grams smoked salmon (flaked)
- One tbsp. olive oil
- One clove of garlic (crushed)
- Two tsps. balsamic vinegar

Method:

1. Start by preheating the oven to 160 degrees Celsius. Use baking paper for lining a baking sheet. Add couscous to the sheet and cook according to the packet instructions.
2. Spread lettuce over a baking tray and spray with oil—Bake for about ten minutes.
3. Place crispy lettuce, couscous, shallot, zucchini, salmon, and sprouts on a platter.
4. Mix garlic, oil, and vinegar in a bowl.
5. Drizzle from the top. Toss gently.

Pad Thai

Total Prep & Cooking Time: 40 minutes
Yields: Four Servings
Nutritional Facts: Calories: 293 | Protein: 26g | Fat: 8.3g | Carbs:
29.2g | Fiber: 10.5g

Ingredients:
- 100 grams of rice stick noodles (thin)
- One tsp. tamarind sauce
- One tbsp. tamari
- One tbsp. lemon juice
- One tsp. brown sugar
- 300 grams tofu (firm, cut into pieces of 1.5 cm)
- 200 grams prawns (peeled)
- One white onion (sliced)
- Three cloves of garlic (crushed)
- One red capsicum (sliced)
- One bunch broccolini
- 350 grams carrots (cut into noodle-like shape)
- One cup bean sprouts
- Two tbsps. peanuts (for serving)

Method:
1. Take a large bowl and soak the noodles in boiling water for three minutes.
2. Mix tamari, tamarind, sugar, and lemon juice in a bowl.
3. Take a wok and heat oil in it over a high flame. Stir-fry the pieces of tofu for two minutes. Keep it aside.
4. Spray the wok with oil and add prawns to it—Cook for four minutes.
5. Spray the wok with oil once more and add onions to it. Fry for about two minutes. Add garlic, broccolini, and carrots—Cook for four minutes.
6. Add capsicum and stir-fry for one minute.
7. Add prawns, sauce mixture, and tofu to the wok. Add noodles and toss for two minutes.
8. Serve with peanuts and bean sprouts.

Asparagus, Noodle, and Prawn Salad

Total Prep & Cooking Time: 30 minutes
Yields: Four Servings
Nutritional Facts: Calories: 360 | Protein: 36g | Fat: 13g | Carbs: 36g | Fiber: 8.6g

Ingredients:

- 180 grams soba noodles
- Two bunches of asparagus (diagonally sliced)
- 200 grams snow peas (sliced)
- Two tbsps. tamari
- One tbsp. lemon juice
- Three tsps. sesame oil
- Twp tsps. ginger (grated)
- 500 grams prawns (peeled)
- One clove of garlic (crushed)
- One tbsp. sesame seeds
- One avocado (quartered)
- Three shallots (sliced)

Method:

1. Take a saucepan and cook the noodles in boiling water. Add snow peas and asparagus to the saucepan during the last minutes of cooking. Refresh under running water and drain.
2. Mix tamari, oil, lemon juice, and ginger in a bowl.
3. Take a pan and heat it over a medium flame. Spray the pan with oil and add prawns to it—Cook for two minutes. Stir occasionally.
4. Add garlic to the heated pan and cook for one more minute. Add prawns to the noodle mixture.
5. Take a plate and add sesame seeds to it. Dip the avocado in the seeds for coating.
6. Add shallots and the leftover dressing to the noodle mix. Toss again gently for combining.
7. Serve with avocado from the top.

Fennel and Salmon Salad

Total Prep & Cooking Time: One hour and thirty minutes
Yields: 6 Servings
Nutrition Facts: Calories: 292 | Protein: 27g | Fat: 14g | Carbs: 15g
| Fiber: 7g

Ingredients:
- Four oranges
- One lemon (grated rind)
- Two tbsps. Dijon mustard
- Two tbsps. fresh dill (chopped)
- Three 200 grams fillets of salmon (skinless)
- 250 grams of snow peas (sliced)
- Two fennel bulbs (sliced)
- 150 grams baby spinach
- 120 grams of salad leaves
- One tbsp. balsamic vinegar (white)
- Two tbsps. pistachios (chopped, for serving)

Method:
1. Grate the rind of one orange and then juice. Peel the remaining oranges and cut into rounds.
2. Combine orange rind, lemon rind, half of the orange juice, mustard, and one tbsp. dill in a ceramic dish. Add the fillets of salmon and coat properly. Marinate for one hour in the fridge.
3. Preheat a barbecue on medium. Spray the barbecue with olive oil. Drain the marinade and add the salmon to the barbecue. Cook for three minutes on each side. Flake the salmon coarsely.
4. Soak the snow peas in boiling water for one minute.
5. Take a bowl and combine snow peas, salad leaves, fennel, and slices of orange in a bowl. Whisk mustard, vinegar, dill, and orange juice in another bowl.
6. Add half of the dressing to the salad and toss for combining.
7. Serve the salads on a plate and top it with cooked salmon. Drizzle leftover dressing from the top and sprinkle some pistachios.

Fish Taco and Chipotle Avocado

Total Prep & Cooking Time: 40 minutes
Yields: Four Servings
Nutritional Facts: Calories: 303 | Protein: 27g | Fat: 14g | Carbs: 32g | Fiber: 6g

Ingredients:

- Two tbsps. lime juice
- One tbsp. olive oil
- One tsp. paprika
- One clove of garlic (crushed)
- Two tsps. chipotle sauce
- 400 grams white fish fillets (firm, fish of your choice)
- 200 grams capsicum (deseeded, halved)
- Two zucchini (cut into discs)
- Half avocado
- One butter lettuce
- Eight corn tortillas (warmed)
- Coriander leaves (for serving)

Method:

1. Mix one tbsp. lime juice, paprika, oil, one tsp. chipotle, and garlic in a shallow dish. Add the fillets of fish and coat properly. Marinate for ten minutes.
2. Preheat a barbecue grill or chargrill. Spray zucchini, capsicum, and the fillets of fish with oil.
3. Cook zucchini and capsicum for two minutes or until soft.
4. Cook the fish fillets for two minutes on both sides for two minutes or until browned.
5. Process lime juice, avocado, and chipotle in a blender. Make a fine paste.
6. Divide grilled veggies, lettuce, and fish among the warmed tortillas.
7. Top the tortillas with a dollop of avocado chipotle.
8. Serve with coriander leaves from the top.

Baked Fish With Parmesan Crumb

Total Prep & Cooking Time: 30 minutes
Yields: Four Servings
Nutritional Facts: Calories: 220 | Protein: 36g | Fat: 6g | Carbs: 3g
| Fiber: 3g

Ingredients:

- Half cup breadcrumbs (multi-grain)
- One-fourth cup parsley (chopped)
- One-third cup parmesan cheese (grated)
- One tsp. lemon rind (grated)
- One tsp. olive oil
- Four thick fish steaks (white)
- Cooking spray (olive oil)
- Green beans (steamed, for serving)
- Boiled potatoes (for serving)

Method:

1. Preheat your oven to 200 degrees Celsius. Mix parsley, breadcrumbs, lemon rind, parmesan, pepper, and salt in a mixing bowl. Drizzle some oil.
2. Press the mixture of breadcrumbs on the flesh-side of the fish fillets for making an even topping.
3. Take a baking tray and place the fish skin-side down. Spray some oil. Bake for about fifteen minutes or until the crumbs are golden in color.
4. Serve with potatoes and steamed beans.

Vietnamese Rice Noodle and Prawn Salad

Total Prep & Cooking Time: 45 minutes
Yields: Four Servings
Nutritional Facts: Calories: 301 | Protein: 22g | Fat: 1.6g | Carbs: 42g | Fiber: 3.9g

Ingredients:

- 200 grams of rice noodles
- One carrot (cut like matchsticks)
- One cucumber (cut like matchsticks)
- One red chili (cut like matchsticks)
- 300 grams prawns (peeled, cooked)
- One cup of bean sprouts
- Half cup basil leaves
- One-fourth cup coriander leaves
- One-third cup mint leaves

For dressing:

- Two tbsps. brown sugar
- Three tbsps. fish sauce
- 80 ml of lime juice
- One red chili (chopped)
- One clove of garlic (chopped)

Method:

1. For the dressing, mix fish sauce, juice of lime, and sugar in a small bowl. Add garlic and chili. Stir well.
2. Prepare the noodles following the instructions on the packet. Drain and keep to the side.
3. Add cucumber, carrot, prawns, chili, herbs, and bean sprouts to the noodles bowl. Add the prepared dressing and toss properly for combining.

Fish Fajitas With Avocado and Bean Salsa

Total Prep & Cooking Time: 30 minutes
Yields: Four Servings
Nutritional Facts: Calories: 346 | Protein: 38g | Fat: 11.3g | Carbs:
28g | Fiber: 13.3g

Ingredients:

- Two tsps. paprika (sweet)
- Half tsp. chili flakes
- 600 grams fillets of white fish (firm)
- 400 grams canned black beans (rinsed)
- Half ripe avocado (sliced)
- Twelve grape tomatoes
- One red chili (chopped)
- One tbsp. lime juice
- Two tsp. olive oil
- Half cup yogurt (low-fat)
- Two tsp. chipotle sauce
- Eight corn tortillas (chargrilled)
- Four radishes (sliced)

Method:

1. Mix chili flakes and paprika in a bowl. Sprinkle the spice mix on the fillets of fish.
2. Preheat a skillet over a high flame. Cook the fillets of fish for three minutes on both sides.
3. Take a large bowl and combine black beans, chili, tomato, avocado, olive oil, and lime juice. Season with pepper and salt.
4. Combine chipotle sauce and yogurt in a bowl.
5. Break the fillets of fish into big chunks. Divide the tortillas among plates and top with radish, fish, a dollop of yogurt chipotle, and black bean salsa.

Kale, Mushroom, and Salmon Noodle Bowl

Total Prep & Cooking Time: One hour and twenty minutes
Yields: Four Servings
Nutritional Facts: Calories: 365 | Protein: 32g | Fat: 17g | Carbs: 38g | Fiber: 7.3g

Ingredients:

- One tsp. wasabi paste
- Two tbsps. soy sauce
- Two tbsps. mirin
- One tsp. ginger (grated)
- Two fillets of salmon (skinless)
- One tbsp. olive oil (extra virgin)
- 400 grams of mixed mushrooms (quartered)
- One red capsicum (cut in strips)
- One clove of garlic (crushed)
- 100 grams kale (chopped)
- 170 grams soba noodles

Method:

1. Mix soy sauce, wasabi, ginger, and mirin in a small bowl. Pour half of the mixture in a shallow dish and add fillets of salmon. Coat well and marinate for one hour.
2. Preheat a grill pan over high heat. Lightly spray some oil on the pan. Grill the fish fillets for three minutes on both sides or until properly cooked. Flake the fillets.
3. Take a frying pan and add three tsps. oil to it. Cook mushrooms for about two minutes or until they turn golden.
4. Heat rest of the oil in the pan and add capsicum and garlic— Cook for about two minutes. Start adding the kale and cook until the kale wilts.
5. Cook the noodles in hot boiling water for reaching al dente.
6. Divide the mushroom, noodles, salmon, and kale mixture among serving bowls.
7. Drizzle leftover marinade from the top.

Smoked Salmon Salad and Green Dressing

Total Prep & Cooking Time: 35 minutes
Yields: Four Servings
Nutritional Facts: Calories: 260 | Protein: 21g | Fat: 12g | Carbs: 19g | Fiber: 9.2g

Ingredients:

- Half cup green lentils (rinsed)
- Two bulbs of fennel (sliced)
- Half cup yogurt
- Two tbsps. parsley (chopped)
- Three tbsps. chives (chopped)
- One tbsp. tarragon (chopped)
- One tbsp. baby capers (rinsed)
- One tsp. lemon rind (grated)
- One red onion (sliced)
- One tbsp. lemon juice
- 70 grams baby spinach
- Half avocado (sliced)
- 180 grams smoked salmon

Method:

1. Start by cooking the lentils in a saucepan in boiling water— Cook for twenty minutes or until soft.
2. Heat a grill pan and spray some oil. Add fennel slices and cook for two minutes.
3. Process parsley, yogurt, tarragon, chives, lemon rind, and capers in a food processor. Make a fine mix.
4. Add onion, sugar, lemon juice, and some salt in a bowl.
5. Combine fennel, lentils, spinach, onion mix, and avocado in a bowl. Divide the mix among plates.
6. Top the salad with salmon. Add lentils by the side and drizzle with the green dressing.

Healthy Pasta Salmon Bake

Total Prep & Cooking Time: 45 minutes
Yields: 6 Servings
Nutrition Facts: Calories: 331 | Protein: 25g | Fat: 10g | Carbs: 35g | Fiber: 11g

Ingredients:

- 300 grams penne pasta
- 500 grams cauliflower florets
- One tbsp. olive oil
- One onion (chopped)
- Two cloves of garlic (crushed)
- Two 400 grams cans of cherry tomatoes
- Two tsps. vinegar (balsamic)
- 500 grams of canned red salmon (flaked)
- 70 grams baby spinach
- 100 grams ricotta (crumbled)
- 20 grams parmesan (shredded)

Method:

1. Preheat your oven at 180 degrees Celsius.
2. Cook the pasta in a pan of boiling water for ten minutes. Add florets of cauliflower to the water during the last two minutes.
3. Heat oil in a pan over a medium flame. Add onions to the pan and cook for five minutes. Add tomato, garlic, and vinegar—Cook for six minutes.
4. Combine pasta, tomato mixture, cauliflower, spinach, and salmon in a baking dish. Sprinkle cheese from the top.
5. Bake for twenty minutes.

Zucchini Tuna Noodle Bake

Total Prep & Cooking Time: 60 minutes
Yields: 6 Servings
Nutrition Facts: Calories: 165 | Protein: 17g | Fat: 6g | Carbs: 0g |
Fiber: 3g

Ingredients:

- Four zucchini (cut like noodles)
- Two tsps. olive oil
- Half yellow onion (diced)
- Two cans of flaked tuna
- One tbsp. tomato paste
- One can diced tomatoes
- Half cup skimmed milk
- Half tsp. kosher salt
- One tsp thyme
- One-fourth tsp. black pepper (ground)
- Half cup cheddar cheese (fat-free, shredded)
- One-fourth cup parmesan (fat-free, shredded)

Method:

1. Preheat your oven at 200 degrees Celsius.
2. Spray a pan with cooking spray. Spread the zucchini noodles in a layer.
3. Take a skillet and heat oil in it over a medium flame. Start adding onions to the oil. Cook the onions for three minutes. Add tomato paste and tuna. Cook for one minute.
4. Add diced tomatoes, thyme, milk, pepper, and salt. Simmer the mixture and add parmesan. Allow the cheese to melt.
5. Pour the mix of tuna over the noodles of zucchini. Sprinkle cheddar from the top and bake for twenty minutes or until the cheese melts.

Coconut Mussels Curry

Total Prep & Cooking Time: 50 minutes
Yields: Four Servings
Nutritional Facts: Calories: 310 | Protein: 30g | Fat: 17g | Carbs: 12g | Fiber: 3.6g

Ingredients:

- Two tbsps. of water
- Half cup onion (diced)
- Half cup red capsicum (diced)
- Three cloves of garlic (minced)
- Half tsp. black pepper (ground)
- Two tbsps. curry powder
- One cup of coconut milk
- Half cup of vegetable broth
- Two pounds mussels (washed)
- Half cup cilantro (chopped)

Method:

1. Take a skillet and add water to it. Heat the water and add capsicum, onion, and garlic. Cook until the onions turn soft. Add more water if needed.
2. Add curry powder, pepper, coconut milk, and broth. Stir well. Simmer the mixture and add mussels.
3. Cover the skillet and cook for about five minutes or until the mussels open.
4. Serve with cilantro from the top.

Stir-fried Honey Garlic Shrimp

Total Prep & Cooking Time: 30 minutes
Yields: Four Servings
Nutritional Facts: Calories: 290 | Protein: 30g | Fat: 4g | Carbs: 31g
| Fiber: 7g

Ingredients:

- One tbsp. coconut oil
- One pound shrimp (peeled)
- Two cloves of garlic (minced)
- One tbsp. ginger (minced)
- One small onion (cut in strips)
- One red capsicum (cut in strips)
- One cup peas
- Half tsp. salt
- Two tbsp. honey
- One tbsp. soy sauce
- Half tbsp. orange zest

Method:

1. Take a skillet and add oil to it. After the oil gets hot, add half of the ginger, half of the garlic, and shrimp. Cook for five minutes and keep aside.
2. In the same skillet, add onion, peas, capsicum, and the leftover ginger and garlic. Cook for five minutes or until the veggies get soft.
3. Add the shrimp to the pan and season with pepper, salt, soy sauce, honey, and zest of orange.
4. Toss properly and serve hot.

Seared Tuna and Fennel-Orange Olive Salsa

Total Prep & Cooking Time: Twenty minutes
Yields: 2 Servings
Nutritional Facts: Calories: 375 | Protein: 51g | Fat: 12g | Carbs: 13g
| Fiber: 6.5g

Ingredients:

- Two fillets of tuna
- Two tsps. cumin (ground)
- 400 grams of fennel (remove the cores, diced)
- Half cup kalamata olives (chopped)
- One tsp. olive oil
- One orange
- Kosher salt

Method:

1. Take a skillet and heat it over a high flame. Season the fillets of tuna with salt, cumin, and pepper. Place the fillets in the skillet. Sear the fish on both sides.
2. Cool the fish for three minutes and slice thinly with the help of a sharp knife.
3. Add olive oil and fennel in a skillet over a low flame. Cook fennel until soft. Combine the cooked fennel with orange segments and olives. Add pepper and salt according to taste.
4. Serve the seared fish with salsa on the top.

Salmon With Asparagus and Polenta

Total Prep & Cooking Time: 40 minutes
Yields: 2 Servings
Nutrition Facts: Calories: 390 | Protein: 30g | Fat: 3.2g | Carbs: 23g
| Fiber: 9.3g

Ingredients:
- Half cup of cornmeal (ground)
- Two tsps. olive oil (extra virgin)
- One clove of garlic (minced)
- One tsp. thyme (fresh)
- Two tsps. of salt
- Two cups of water
- One cup of sun-dried tomatoes (chopped finely)
- One-third cup parmesan cheese (grated)
- 450 grams of salmon fillet (divide into two equal pieces)
- Three tsps. of lemon zest
- One-fourth tsp. black pepper (ground)
- 400 grams of asparagus (cut in two-inch pieces)
- One lime (juiced)

Method:
1. Combine olive oil, cornmeal, thyme, garlic, water, and one-fourth tsp. of salt in a microwave-safe bowl. Microwave the mix for three minutes.
2. Stir the mixture and reheat for three minutes until the polenta thickens. Add cheese and sun-dried tomatoes to the mixture. Cover the bowl and keep it aside.
3. Take a baking dish. Start adding the fish with the skin-side down. Season the fish with pepper, salt, and zest of lemon.
4. Cover the dish with the help of a wax paper.
5. Microwave the fish for three minutes on high setting. Check once if the fish is cooked evenly. Microwave for another thirty seconds if needed.
6. Place the cut asparagus in a bowl with one tbsp. of water. Microwave for two minutes and season with lemon juice and salt.
7. Serve the fish with polenta and asparagus by the side.

Snapper Taco With Salsa

Total Prep & Cooking Time: 30 minutes
Yields: 2 Servings
Nutrition Facts: Calories: 400 | Protein: 39g | Fat: 1.2g | Carbs: 28g
| Fiber: 5.6g

Ingredients:

- 450 grams of snapper fillet
- Black pepper (ground)
- Cracked kosher salt
- Four tortillas (corn)
- Cooking spray

For salad:

- On avocado (peeled, diced)
- One cup of grape tomatoes (halved)
- Two tbsps. chives
- Half juice of a lime

Method:

1. Take a grill pan and heat it over a high flame.
2. Cut some slits on the fillets of the fish. Season with pepper and salt. Coat the fish with cooking spray.
3. Add the fish to the grill and cook for about ten minutes or until grilled properly. Flip the fish and cook for another ten minutes. Make sure that the fish is flaky and white.
4. Place corn tortillas on the grill and heat until charred.
5. For the salsa, mix grape tomatoes, avocado, lime juice, and chives in a bowl. Season according to taste. Toss well for combining.
6. Divide the cooked fish among the tortillas and top with the salsa.

CHAPTER 6:
RECIPES FOR BEEF AND PORK

If you are thinking that you will not be able to consume red meat while being on a diet, then you are completely wrong. There are various beef and pork meal recipes that you can include in your Sirtfood Diet plan.

Beef Noodle Salad With Miso Roast Pumpkin

Total Prep & Cooking Time: 45 minutes
Yields: Four Servings
Nutritional Facts: Calories: 375 | Protein: 30g | Fat: 7g | Carbs: 42g | Fiber: 9.2g

Ingredients:

- One large pumpkin (cut in wedges, deseeded)
- One-fourth cup of mirin seasoning
- Two tbsps. miso paste (white)
- One tbsp. vinegar (rice wine)
- One and a half tsps. wasabi paste
- One tsp. honey
- 100 grams soba noodles
- 350 grams beef fillet steak
- 200 grams of peas
- 50 grams pea sprouts
- One-fourth cup ginger (pickled)
- Two shallots (sliced)

Method:

1. Preheat your oven to 180 degrees Celsius. Take a baking tray and line it with baking paper.
2. Place pumpkin on the tray and spray with some oil. Roast for about ten minutes.

3. Take a bowl and whisk miso, mirin, wasabi, honey, and vinegar. Drizzle half of the mixture over the roasted pumpkin. Roast again for twenty minutes.
4. Cook the noodles in boiling water.
5. Heat a pan over medium flame. Spray the steak with oil and cook for five minutes. Season.
6. Drizzle twp tsp. of the dressing and cook for two more minutes.
7. Add sprouts, peas, shallot, ginger, and cooked beef to the prepared noodles.
8. Add the remaining dressing and toss.
9. Place the roasted pumpkins on a plate and top with the noodle salad.

Asian Slaw With Crumbed Pork

Total Prep & Cooking Time: 45 minutes
Yields: Four Servings
Nutritional Facts: Calories: 302 | Protein: 36g | Fat: 14g | Carbs: 9g
| Fiber: 8g

Ingredients:

- Three-fourth cup almond meal
- Two tsps. lime rind (grated)
- Half cup coriander (chopped)
- Two red chilies (chopped)
- Two egg whites
- Four 135 grams of pork steaks (lean loin)
- Half cup red cabbage (shredded)
- One bunch of buk choy (shredded)
- One apple (sliced)
- Half cup of mint leaves (torn)
- Two tbsps. lime juice
- Twp tsps. olive oil
- Half tsp. caster sugar

Method:

1. Mix lime rind, almond meal, half of chopped chili, and coriander in a dish.
2. Whisk the egg whites in another bowl.
3. Coat the steaks in egg white and then dip it in almond meal mixture for coating properly. Keep the steaks in the fridge for ten minutes.
4. Take a skillet and heat it over a medium flame. Add olive oil to the pan. Cook the coated pork steaks for three minutes on each side until golden in color.
5. Combine buk choy, cabbage, mint, apple, and coriander in a bowl. Add olive oil, sugar, and lime juice in another bowl. Add the dressing to the prepared slaw and toss well.
6. Divide the pork steaks and slaw among plates and serve.

Healthy Beef Chowmein

Total Prep & Cooking Time: 40 minutes
Yields: 6 Servings
Nutrition Facts: Calories: 360 | Protein: 29g | Fat: 10.2g | Carbs: 42g | Fiber: 10.4g

Ingredients:
- 350 grams chowmein noodles
- Two tsps. cornflour
- Two tbsps. soy sauce
- One tbsp. oyster sauce
- One cube of beef stock
- One tbsp. vegetable oil
- 500 grams of beef mince (lean)
- One bunch of pak choy
- One onion (cut in wedges)
- One stalk of celery (sliced)
- Two cloves of garlic (crushed)
- Two carrots (cut in strips)
- 100 grams of snow peas
- 450 grams of baby corn (halved)
- Two red chilies (sliced)

Method:
1. Start by cooking the noodles in boiling water.
2. Combine soy sauce and cornflour in a bowl. Add the stock cube, oyster sauce, and half a cup of water. Combine well.
3. Take a pan and heat it over a medium flame. Add oil to the pan. Add the beef mince and stir-fry for five minutes until browned.
4. Add pak choy to the frying pan and cook until the leaves wilt. Add celery and onion along with garlic. Stir-fry for five minutes.
5. Add the beef mince to the pan and combine well.
6. Add sauce mix, snow peas, and carrot to the pan and cook until the sauce thickens. Add the cooked noodles and toss for combining.
7. Serve with pak choy and chilies from the top.

Bean and Beef Stir-fry

Total Prep & Cooking Time: Twenty minutes
Yields: Four Servings
Nutritional Facts: Calories: 260 | Protein: 33g | Fat: 7g | Carbs: 15g
| Fiber: 6g

Ingredients:

- Three cloves of garlic (sliced)
- 500 grams of beef mince (lean)
- Two tbsps. Thai seasoning
- One cup of pineapple juice
- One tbsp. oyster sauce
- Two tsps. coconut sugar
- 350 grams of green beans (sliced)
- One cup coriander (chopped)
- Half cup mint leaves (chopped)
- Two red chilies (sliced)

Method:

1. Heat a large skillet over a medium flame. Add oil to the skillet. Add garlic to the pan and cook for two minutes. Remove the garlic and add beef to the skillet. Cook the beef for five minutes. Make sure the beef is brown in color.
2. Add the seasoning and stir for one minute. Add oyster sauce, juice, and sugar. Simmer the mix for ten minutes and stir occasionally until the liquid turns sticky.
3. Add beans to the pan and cook for two minutes. Add mint and coriander.
4. Serve with garlic and chili from the top.

Beef Stir-Fry With Peanuts and Broccoli

Total Prep & Cooking Time: 30 minutes
Yields: Four Servings
Nutritional Facts: Calories: 319 | Protein: 36g | Fat: 9g | Carbs: 32g
| Fiber: 12g

Ingredients:

- Two tsps. fish sauce
- One tbsp. lime juice
- One tsp. brown sugar
- Two tsps. peanut oil
- 500 grams of beef mince (lean)
- One red onion (chopped)
- Two cloves of garlic (crushed)
- Two tsps. ginger (grated)
- Two red chilies (chopped)
- 400 grams of eggplant (cut in pieces of 2 cm)
- 350 grams of broccoli florets
- One bunch pay choy
- Two tbsps. peanuts (chopped, for serving)

Method:

1. Add lime juice, sugar along with in a bowl. Stir well for dissolving the sugar.
2. Heat a frying pan and add oil in it. Add the beef and stir-fry for four minutes. Keep aside.
3. Heat the leftover oil in the pan and start adding onion to it. Cook for two minutes and add ginger, chili, and garlic. Stir-fry for one minute.
4. Add eggplant, broccoli, and water to the pan. Stir-fry for three minutes or until tender. Add the pak choy and cook for one minute.
5. Add the cooked beef to the pan along with the fish sauce mix. Combine well.
6. Serve with peanuts from the top.

Grilled Steak and Smoky White Bean Mash

Total Prep & Cooking Time: 30 minutes
Yields: 6 Servings
Nutrition Facts: Calories: 345 | Protein: 39g | Fat: 17g | Carbs: 12g
| Fiber: 13g

Ingredients:

- One cauliflower (cut in florets)
- Half cup olive oil
- Two sprigs of rosemary (chopped)
- Three cloves of garlic (crushed)
- One lemon (half rind, half juiced)
- 400 grams of canned beans (cannellini, rinsed)
- Half cup of water
- Two 300 grams beef steaks

Method:

1. Heat a chargrill on medium. Place the florets of cauliflower in a bowl and drizzle some oil on it. Toss for coating. Grill for ten minutes or until tender.
2. Take a saucepan and heat it over medium flame. Add one tbsp. oil to the pan and add garlic, lemon rind, and rosemary—Cook for thirty seconds. Add beans, lemon, juice, and water to the pan—Cook for four minutes. Add cauliflower to the mixture. Cook the mixture for five minutes. Use a blender for processing the mixture until smooth.
3. Drizzle some oil on the steaks and cook for five minutes. Slice the steaks after cooling.
4. Divide the prepared mash among the plates and top them with steaks.

Celeriac Mash With Balsamic Pork

Total Prep & Cooking Time: 2 hours 30 minutes
Yields: Four Servings
Nutritional Facts: Calories: 360 | Protein: 38g | Fat: 12g | Carbs: 22g | Fiber: 11g

Ingredients:
- 700 grams of pork fillet
- Two onions (sliced)
- Four cloves of garlic
- Two tsps. fennel seeds
- Two tsps. rosemary (chopped)
- Two and a half tbsps. balsamic vinegar
- One cup of chicken stock
- 350 grams of potatoes (chopped)
- Two tbsps. milk (warmed)
- Three tbsps. parsley (chopped)
- One red chili (chopped)
- Two tsps. lemon rind (grated)

Method:
1. Preheat your oven to 140 degrees Celsius. Spray a casserole dish with oil and add pork to it. Cook the pork for five minutes or until brown in color. Keep aside.
2. Take a frying pan and add oil in it. Add garlic, onion, rosemary, and fennel after the oil gets hot. Cook for five minutes and add vinegar. Simmer the mixture for one minute. Add chicken stock to the pan, along with half a cup of water. Bring the mixture to a boil.
3. Add the mixture to the pork dish and bake for about two hours covered.
4. Shred the pork.
5. Cook potato in a pan with boiling water for ten minutes. Drain the water and add milk. Mash the potatoes until smooth and season with salt.
6. Mix chili, parsley, and rind in a small bowl. Divide the prepared mash among plates and top with pork.

Veggie Beef Pie

Total Prep & Cooking Time: Three hours and thirty minutes
Yields: Eight Servings
Nutrition Facts: Calories: 310 | Protein: 37g | Fat: 15g | Carbs: 17g
| Fiber: 9.6g

Ingredients:

- Two tbsps. olive oil (extra virgin)
- One kg beef steak (cut in pieces of 3 cm)
- 200 grams mushrooms (halved)
- One onion (chopped)
- Two cloves of garlic (chopped)
- Two carrots (chopped)
- One zucchini (chopped)
- 400 grams canned tomatoes (chopped)
- One cup of water
- Three sprigs of thyme
- 500 grams of cauliflower florets
- 400 grams lentils (rinsed)
- One cup peas (frozen)
- Five pastry sheets

Method:

1. Heat oil in a pan and cook the beef. Cook for four minutes and keep aside.
2. Add remaining oil to the pan and cook the mushrooms for five minutes. Keep aside.
3. Add garlic, onion, zucchini, and carrot to the pan—Cook for ten minutes. Add beef to the pan. Mix well. Add tomato and water to the pan. Boil the mixture. Reduce the flame and simmer for two hours.
4. Add lentils, cauliflower, and mushrooms and cook for twenty minutes. Cook until the liquid reduces. Add the peas and season.
5. Preheat your oven at 160 degrees Celsius.

6. Transfer the mixture of beef to a deep pie dish. Spray one pastry sheet with olive oil and place over the mixture of beef. Repeat with the other sheets and tuck in the dish edges for sealing. Spray with olive oil from the top.
7. Bake for forty minutes.

Pork Bake and Roast Mushroom

Total Prep & Cooking Time: 45 minutes
Yields: Four Servings
Nutritional Facts: Calories: 310 | Protein: 40g | Fat: 12g | Carbs: 16g | Fiber: 7g

Ingredients:

- 500 grams of baby potatoes (halved)
- Two tbsps. lemon juice
- Two cloves of garlic (sliced)
- Two tsps. Dijon mustard
- Two tbsps. olive oil (extra virgin)
- 400 grams of mixed mushrooms
- Three shallots (sliced)
- Eight sprigs of thyme
- 600 grams of pork fillet (cut in pieces of 4 cm)
- Half cup parmesan (grated)

Method:

1. Preheat your oven at 190 degrees Celsius. Place the potatoes in a bowl and microwave for five minutes.
2. Combine garlic, lemon juice, mustard, and one tbsp. oil in a bowl. Add potatoes and mushrooms in a roasting pan. Sprinkle thyme, shallot, and lemon mixture from the top. Roast for fifteen minutes. Make sure the ingredients are soft.
3. Heat rest of the oil in a pan over medium flame. Season the fillet of pork and cook for two minutes.
4. Add cooked pork to the roasting pan. Add parmesan from the top. Roast for another ten minutes. Rest the dish for three minutes.
5. Serve with thyme from the top.

Quinoa, Lentil, and Apple Salad With Maple Pork

Total Prep & Cooking Time: 35 minutes
Yields: Four Servings
Nutritional Facts: Calories: 306 | Protein: 32g | Fat: 5g | Carbs: 35g | Fiber: 8.6g

Ingredients:

- Two small apples (cut in wedges)
- One red onion (cut in wedges)
- Two tsps. olive oil (extra virgin)
- Two tbsps. lemon juice
- One tbsp. maple syrup
- One tbsp. water
- Half tsp. chili flakes
- 450 grams of pork fillet
- Half cup quinoa (rinsed)
- Three-fourth cup of water
- 400 grams canned brown lentils (rinsed)
- Half cup parsley (chopped)
- Half cup mint (chopped)
- Two sticks of celery (cut like matchsticks)

Method:

1. Preheat your oven at 160 degrees Celsius.
2. Use baking paper for lining a baking tray. Place the apples on the tray. Drizzle some oil. Toss for combining. Roast for twenty minutes.
3. Combine half of the lemon juice, water, syrup, chili, and water in a bowl.
4. Heat a frying pan over medium flame. Spray the fillet of pork with oil. Cook for five minutes.
5. Pour the lemon mixture on the fillet and roast for ten minutes. Slice the pork and allow the juices of the pan to thicken.

6. Add water and quinoa to a small pan over medium flame. Boil the mixture. Simmer the mixture for ten minutes or until the quinoa is tender.
7. Combine apple mixture, quinoa, lentils, mint, parsley, lemon juice, and celery in a bowl. Season with pepper and salt.
8. Divide among serving plates and top with cooked pork. Drizzle pan juices from the top.

Pumpkin and Pork With Chimichurri

Total Prep & Cooking Time: 45 minutes
Yields: Four Servings
Nutritional Facts: Calories: 350 | Protein: 32g | Fat: 18g | Carbs: 14g | Fiber: 8g

Ingredients:

- One kg pumpkin (cut in wedges)
- 500 grams of pork fillet (lean)
- Half cup almonds (chopped)
- 40 grams arugula

For Chimichurri:

- One red chili (chopped)
- Two cloves of garlic (crushed)
- One cup coriander leaves (chopped)
- Half cup parsley (chopped)
- Half cup of mint leaves
- One-fourth cup of red wine vinegar
- Two tbsps. olive oil

Method:

1. Preheat your oven to 200 degrees Celsius.
2. Use baking paper for lining two baking trays. Place the pumpkin on the trays. Spray with some oil—Bake for half an hour.
3. Spray the fillet of pork with oil. Season the pork.
4. Heat a pan over medium flame and cook the pork for five minutes.
5. For preparing the chimichurri, add garlic, chili, parsley, coriander, vinegar, and mint in a food processor. Process until chopped finely. Add olive oil to the mixture and stir.
6. Slice the pork fillet thickly. Arrange the pork with the pumpkin on serving plates. Top with almond, arugula, and chimichurri sauce from the top.

Pork With Orange Glaze and Snow Pea Salad

Total Prep & Cooking Time: 35 minutes
Yields: Four Servings
Nutritional Facts: Calories: 302 | Protein: 45g | Fat: 9g | Carbs:
8.2g | Fiber: 7.1g

Ingredients:

- Half cup orange juice
- One tbsp. brown sugar
- Two tsps. ginger (grated)
- Four 200 grams cutlets of pork loin
- Two cups of baby peas (frozen)
- Four small-sized radishes (sliced)
- 70 grams feta (crumbled)
- Two tsps. balsamic vinegar (white)
- Two tsps. olive oil

Method:

1. Preheat your oven at 180 degrees Celsius.
2. Take a saucepan. Add sugar, orange juice, and ginger over medium flame. Boil the mixture. Reduce the flame and simmer the mixture for three minutes or until reduced.
3. Take a skillet and heat it over high flame. Add olive oil to the pan—Cook the pork two minutes.
4. Place one wire rack over a baking tray. Line the tray with baking paper. Transfer the cooked pork to the rack. Brush the pork with prepared orange glaze.
5. Roast for fifteen minutes or until the pork is properly cooked.
6. Blanch peas in boiling water until soft and crisp. Wash under cold water.
7. Place radish, peas, and feta in a bowl. Mix olive oil and vinegar and drizzle over the prepared salad. Toss for combining.
8. Divide the salad among serving plates. Serve the glazed pork on top of the salad.

Low-Calorie Pork Chops

Total Prep & Cooking Time: 50 minutes
Yields: Four Servings
Nutritional Facts: Calories: 250 | Protein: 24g | Fat: 9.7g | Carbs: 12g | Fiber: 3g

Ingredients:

- Four pork chops
- Two tsp. cayenne
- One tbsp. butter
- Two tbsp. flour
- One cup chicken stock
- Half cup buttermilk (low-fat)
- One tsp. Dijon mustard

Method:

1. Season the pork chops with cayenne, pepper, and salt. Keep in the refrigerator for one hour.
2. Take a skillet and heat butter in it. Dust the marinated chops with a little bit of flour on both sides.
3. Cook the pork chops for four minutes on each side.
4. Remove the chops from the pan. Add stock, mustard, and buttermilk to the pan. Simmer the mixture for two minutes.
5. Serve the pork chops with buttermilk sauce from the top.

Low-Fat Pork Tenderloin and Pineapple Salsa

Total Prep & Cooking Time: 50 minutes
Yields: Four Servings
Nutritional Facts: Calories: 206 | Protein: 29g | Fat: 9g | Carbs: 21g
| Fiber: 6.3g

Ingredients:

- One tbsp. mustard (Dijon)
- Half tbsp. honey
- 400 grams of pork tenderloin
- Half tbsp. chili powder
- Four slices of pineapple
- One onion (minced)
- Half cup of cilantro (chopped)
- One jalapeno pepper (chopped)
- Four tbsps. lime juice

Method:

1. Preheat a chargrill or barbecue grill.
2. Mix honey, mustard, salt, chili powder, and pepper in a bowl. Rub the honey mixture all over the pork.
3. Place the pineapple slices and the pork on the grill. Grill the pork for ten minutes, turning in between. Make sure that the pork is charred lightly. Grill the pineapple for three minutes on each side.
4. Allow the pork to sit for five minutes.
5. Chop the grilled pineapple slices into small pieces. Mix with jalapeno, onion, lime juice, and cilantro.
6. Slice the pork.
7. Serve with salsa by the side.

Fiery Jerk Pork

Total Prep & Cooking Time: One hour and thirty minutes
Yields: Four Servings
Nutrition Facts: Calories: 220 | Protein: 20g | Fat: 11g | Carbs: 36g | Fiber: 6.8g

Ingredients:

- Two habanero peppers (chopped)
- Eight scallions (chopped)
- Two limes (juiced)
- Two tbsp. of canola oil
- Three cloves of garlic (chopped)
- One tsp. of allspice
- Half tsp. nutmeg
- 400 grams pork loin

Method:

1. Add peppers, lime juice, scallions, garlic, oil, nutmeg, allspice, and a little bit of pepper and salt in a blender. Pulse the ingredients for making a fine paste. You can add some water if the paste is too dry.
2. Marinate the pork with the prepared spice paste. Refrigerate for one hour.
3. Preheat a chargrill or grill pan. Add some oil to the pan and cook the pork. Cook for ten minutes on both sides.

Thai Pork Kebab

Total Prep & Cooking Time: 40 minutes
Yields: 8 Servings
Nutrition Facts: Calories: 220 | Protein: 28g | Fat: 17g | Carbs: 37g
| Fiber: 5.2g

Ingredients:

- Half cup coconut milk
- Two tbsps. Thai curry paste
- One tbsp. of peanut butter
- 400 grams pork loin (cut into three cm pieces)
- One red capsicum (chopped in cubes)
- One red onion (chopped in cubes)
- Eight skewers

Method:

1. Start by preheating the grill pan.
2. Mix curry paste, coconut milk, and peanut butter in a bowl.
3. Keep half of the mix in another bowl.
4. Thread the capsicum, pork, and onion into the skewers. Alternate between veggies and meat.
5. Brush the skewers with the paste.
6. Add the kebab skewers to preheated pan. Cook for four minutes on each side.
7. Serve by brushing the skewers with the remaining curry paste.

Lean Pork Chops and Honey Balsamic Glaze

Total Prep & Cooking Time: One hour and thirty minutes
Yields: Four Servings
Nutrition Facts: Calories: 270 | Protein: 24g | Fat: 17g | Carbs: 32g
| Fiber: 7g

Ingredients:

- Half cup vinegar (balsamic)
- Two tbsps. butter
- One tsp. rosemary (chopped)
- Three tbsps. honey
- Half tsp. pepper flakes
- Four pork chops (thick-cut)

Method:

1. Add butter, honey, vinegar, pepper flakes, and rosemary in a pan. Cook over low flame until the butter melts.
2. Preheat your grill pan or grill.
3. Reserve two tbsps. of the glaze and marinate the pork chops with the rest of the glaze.
4. Add the chops to the grill and cook for six minutes on both sides. The time for cooking will depend on the thickness of the chops.
5. Serve the pork chops by brushing with the reserved glaze.

Beef Stroganoff

Total Prep & Cooking Time: 50 minutes
Yields: Four Servings
Nutritional Facts: Calories: 395 | Protein: 38g | Fat: 10.3g | Carbs: 35g | Fiber: 8.6g

Ingredients:

- 350 grams of beef steak (cut in strips)
- Two tbps. of white flour
- One tbsp. olive oil (extra virgin)
- One onion (sliced)
- Eight button mushrooms (sliced)
- Two tbsps. of Worcestershire sauce
- One tsp. of lemon juice
- One cup of yogurt (Greek)
- Half tsp. of black pepper (ground)
- One-fourth tsp. salt
- Three tbsps. of parsley (chopped)
- One and a half tsps. of Dijon mustard
- Three-fourth tsp. of paprika
- Two tbsps. of each
  - Tomato puree
  - Cognac or brandy
- Three cups of steamed rice

Method:

1. Place beef and flour in a bowl. Coat the beef in flour evenly.
2. Take a skillet and heat it over a medium flame. Add half of the olive oil and add onions to it. Cook the onions for five minutes. Add paprika and give it a stir. Add the sliced mushrooms and cook the mixture for four minutes. Remove the mixture from the pan and keep it in a bowl.
3. Heat the pan over a high flame. Add oil to the pan. Cook the strips of beef in batches. Season with pepper and salt. Cook the strips of beef for one minute or until browned.

4. Add the mixture of mushrooms and onion to the cooked beef. Give it a stir. Add brandy and Worcestershire sauce to the pan. Mix well and simmer the mixture for five minutes.
5. Add tomato puree, yogurt, and Dijon mustard to the pan. Give the mixture a stir and add parsley along with lemon juice.
6. Serve with steamed rice by the side.

CHAPTER 7:
RECIPES FOR SNACKS
AND DESSERTS

Apart from the meal recipes, snacks and desserts are also important. They can help in mending our sudden hunger while fulfilling the nutritional requirements as well. So, I have included some tasty recipes for snacks and desserts that you can include in your Sirtfood Diet plan.

Spicy Green Tea Smoothie

Total Prep & Cooking Time: 35 minutes
Yields: 2 Servings
Nutrition Facts: Calories: 82 | Protein: 2g | Fat: 0.6g | Carbs: 20g | Fiber: 4g

Ingredients:

- One cup green tea (chilled)
- One tsp. cayenne powder
- Four tbsps. lemon juice
- Two tsps. agave nectar
- One pear (cut in pieces)
- One cup of ice cubes
- Two tbsps. yogurt (fat-free)

Method:

1. Put all the listed ingredients in a high speed blender except for the ice cubes. Blend well.
2. Add ice cubes and give the mixture a pulse.
3. Serve immediately.

Crudites With Herb and White Bean Hummus

Total Prep & Cooking Time: 5 minutes
Yields: 1 Serving
Nutrition Facts: Calories: 150 | Protein: 5g | Fat: 9g | Carbs: 13g |
Fiber: 4g

Ingredients:

- One cup white beans (canned)
- One tbsp. chives (chopped)
- Two tbsps. lemon juice
- Two tsps. olive oil
- Raw veggies such as red and green peppers, broccoli, baby carrots, etc.

Method:

1. Mix chives, beans, oil, and lemon juice in a bowl. Mash the mixture with the help of a fork.
2. Serve the hummus with raw veggies of your choice.

Choco-Dipped Banana Bites

Total Prep & Cooking Time: 20minutes
Yields: 4 Servings
Nutrition Facts: Calories: 180 | Protein: 2g | Fat: 6g | Carbs: 36g |
Fiber: 5g

Ingredients:

- Two tsbps. choco chips (semi-sweet)
- One banana (cut into chunks)

Method:

1. Melt the choco chips in a bowl.
2. Dip the pieces of banana in the melted chocolate.
3. Keep in the freezer for twenty minutes.

Turkey Burgers

Total Prep & Cooking Time: 40 minutes
Yields: Four Servings
Nutritional Facts: Calories: 270 | Protein: 29g | Fat: 11g | Carbs: 27g | Fiber: 3g

Ingredients:

- One pound turkey (ground)
- One clove of garlic (minced)
- Half tsp. paprika
- One-fourth tsp. cumin (ground)
- A pinch of kosher salt
- One tsp. black pepper (ground)
- Four slices of grilled sweet onion
- One cup barbecue sauce
- Four buns (toasted)

Method:

1. Mix garlic, turkey, cumin, and paprika in a bowl.
2. Make four patties from the meat mix. Season with pepper and salt.
3. Heat a pan and cook the patties for five minutes on each side.
4. Serve the buns with barbecue sauce and patty in between.

Light Quinoa Snack

Total Prep & Cooking Time: 5 minutes
Yields: 1 Serving
Nutrition Facts: Calories: 300 | Protein: 13g | Fat: 8g | Carbs: 42g
| Fiber: 9g

Ingredients:

- One cup of quinoa (cooked)
- Half cup black beans (canned)
- One tomato (chopped)
- One scallion (sliced)
- One tsp. olive oil
- Two tsps. lemon juice
- Half tsp. salt

Method:

1. Mix the listed ingredients in a mixing bowl. Toss properly for combining.

Egg Salad Sandwich

Total Prep & Cooking Time: 10 minutes
Yields: 1 Serving
Nutrition Facts: Calories: 350 | Protein: 21g | Fat: 13g | Carbs: 45g | Fiber: 9g

Ingredients:

- Two cooked eggs (chopped)
- Two tbsps. Greek yogurt
- Three tbsps. red capsicum (chopped)
- One-fourth tsp. curry powder
- One tsp. ground pepper
- Half tsp. salt
- Two slices of bread (toasted)
- Half cup spinach
- One orange

Method:

1. Combine yogurt, eggs, curry powder, capsicum, pepper, and salt in a bowl. Mix well.
2. Place spinach leaves on the bread slices and top with the egg mix. Serve with orange by the side.

Fruit Parfait With Greek Yogurt

Total Prep & Cooking Time: 5 minutes
Yields: 1 Serving
Nutrition Facts: Calories: 410 | Protein: 21g | Fat: 13g | Carbs: 60g
| Fiber: 10g

Ingredients:

- One cup Greek yogurt
- Two cups mixed nectarines, peaches, and plums (sliced)
- Half cup of rice cereal (puffed)
- Two tbsps. almonds and walnuts (chopped)
- One tbsp. flaxseed (ground)
- Two tbsps. honey

Method:

1. Take a tall jar and start layering fruits, cereals, flaxseed, nuts, and syrup.
2. Repeat the same process for the remaining ingredients in layers.
3. Refrigerate the jar for eight hours.

Avocado Cups

Total Prep & Cooking Time: Twenty minutes
Yields: 2 Servings
Nutritional Facts: Calories: 90 | Protein: 9g | Fat: 0.6g | Carbs: 10g | Fiber: 7g

Ingredients:

- One avocado
- One tbsp. lime juice
- One tbsp. yogurt or sour cream
- Half tsp. cumin (ground)
- Two tbsps. cilantro (chopped)
- Twelve endive leaves

Method:

1. Peel the avocado and mash it.
2. Mix lime juice, yogurt or sour cream, cumin, and cilantro in a bowl.
3. Add the avocado to the mix.
4. Spoon the prepared mix of avocado into the leaves of endive.
5. Top with cilantro.

Garbanzo Salad

Total Prep & Cooking Time: 35 minutes
Yields: 8 Servings
Nutrition Facts: Calories: 160 | Protein: 6g | Fat: 5g | Carbs: 24g |
Fiber: 6g

Ingredients:

- Three cups of fennel bulbs (chopped)
- Two cups tomato (chopped)
- Oen cup red onion (chopped)
- Half cup basil (chopped)
- One-third cup vinegar (balsamic)
- One tbsp. olive oil
- One tsp. pepper (ground)
- One-fourth tsp. salt
- Four cloves of garlic (minced)
- Two cans of chickpeas (garbanzo)
- Half cup feta cheese (crumbled)

Method:

1. Combine the listed ingredients in a mixing bowl. Do not mix the feta.
2. Toss properly for mixing.
3. Allow the salad to rest for half an hour.
4. Serve with feta from the top.

Oats and Dark Chocolate Clusters

Total Prep & Cooking Time: Ten minutes
Yields: Four Servings
Nutritional Facts: Calories: 160 | Protein: 6g | Fat: 7g | Carbs: 18g
| Fiber: 4g

Ingredients:

- Two tbsps. peanut butter
- Three tbsps. milk (low-fat)
- One-fourth cup choco chips (semi-sweet)
- One cup rolled oats

Method:

1. Start by heating milk, peanut butter, and choco chips in a pan for two minutes over medium flame. Make sure that the choco chips melt completely.
2. Add the rolled oats to the pan. Stir properly. Remove the pan from heat.
3. Take a spoon and make ball-shaped dollops from the mix. Place the balls on a baking sheet. Put in the freezer for five minutes

Crispy Chickpea Slaw

Total Prep & Cooking Time: Ten minutes
Yields: Two Servings
Nutritional Facts: Calories: 330 | Protein: 17g | Fat: 7g | Carbs: 50g
| Fiber: 14g

Ingredients:

- Half cup plain yogurt
- One tbsp. cider vinegar
- Two tbsps. of water
- Half tsp. kosher salt
- One tsp. black pepper (ground)
- One can chickpeas (rinsed)
- Three cups green cabbage (sliced)
- Two stalks of celery (sliced)
- Two carrots (peeled in strips)
- Three tbsps. sesame seeds (toasted)

Method:

1. Take a mixing bowl and add vinegar, yogurt, pepper, salt, and water. Add celery, chickpeas, cabbage, and carrots to the bowl. Toss well for combining. Sprinkle sesame seeds from the top.
2. Transfer the prepared slaw into airtight containers. Keep the container in the refrigerator for five hours.

Sliced Pear and Ham Swiss Sandwich

Total Prep & Cooking Time: 10 minutes
Yields: 1 Serving
Nutrition Facts: Calories: 310 | Protein: 18g | Fat: 10g | Carbs: 52g | Fiber: 10.6g

Ingredients:

- One tbsp. Greek yogurt (low-fat)
- One-fourth tsp. dill (dried)
- Two slices of bread
- One ounce sliced ham (lean)
- One pear (sliced)
- Half cup Swiss cheese (sliced)

Method:

1. Mix dill and yogurt in a bowl. Stir well.
2. Spread the prepared yogurt mix on the slices of bread. Top one slice of bread with half slice of pear, ham, Swiss cheese, and the remaining slices of bread.
3. Serve with leftover pear slices by the side.

Almond Butter and Banana Toast

Total Prep & Cooking Time: 10 minutes
Yields: 1 Serving
Nutrition Facts: Calories: 270 | Protein: 7g | Fat: 11g | Carbs: 40g |
Fiber: 6.5g

Ingredients:

- One tbsp. almond butter
- Two slices of rye bread (toasted)
- One large banana (sliced)

Method:

1. Spread the almond butter on the toasted bread slices.
2. Add banana slices on the top and enjoy!

Lentil Soup and Toasted Pita

Total Prep & Cooking Time: 30 minutes
Yields: Four Servings
Nutritional Facts: Calories: 340 | Protein: 20g | Fat: 5g | Carbs: 52g | Fiber: 23g

Ingredients:

- One tbsp. olive oil (extra virgin)
- Two stalks of celery (chopped)
- Two carrots (peeled, chopped)
- One large onion
- Two cloves of garlic (minced)
- Two tsps. oregano (dried)
- Half tsp. salt
- One tsp. pepper (ground)
- Ten cups of water
- One cup lentils (dried)
- Three tbsps. lemon juice
- Four pitas (whole-wheat, cut in four triangles, toasted)

Method:

1. Take a pan and heat oil in it over a medium flame. Add carrot, celery, garlic, onion, oregano, pepper, and salt to the pan—Cook for about five minutes.
2. Add lentils to the pan along with water. Simmer the mixture for fifteen minutes. Cover the pan.
3. Use a hand blender for pureeing the soup until thick and smooth.
4. Drizzle lemon juice and give it a stir.
5. Serve with pita triangles.

Fudgy Brownies

Total Prep & Cooking Time: Three hours and twenty minutes
Yields: Twenty Servings
Nutritional Facts: Calories: 101 | Protein: 2g | Fat: 3g | Carbs: 16g |
Fiber: 2g

Ingredients:

- Three-fourth cup flour
- Two-third cup sugar
- Three tbsps. cocoa powder (unsweetened)
- Three ounces of chocolate (semi-sweet, chopped)
- Two tbsps. of canola oil
- Half cup of granulated sugar
- Two tbsps. corn syrup (light)
- Two tsps. vanilla extract
- Half tsp. salt
- One egg
- One-third cup walnuts (chopped)

Method:

1. Preheat your oven at 180 degrees Celsius. Use aluminum foil for lining a baking tray. Coat the tray with cooking spray.
2. Take a bowl and sift sugar, cocoa, and flour.
3. Add chocolate in a pan, along with some oil. Heat it over low flame. Allow the chocolate to melt.
4. Add corn syrup, granulated sugar, salt, and vanilla to the chocolate.
5. Add egg to the chocolate mixture. Stir vigorously until the egg combines properly.
6. Add the dry ingredients along with walnuts. Fold the mixture properly and add any remaining chocolate.
7. Add the flour mixture and fold properly.
8. Add the brownie mixture to the baking tray and bake for twenty minutes. Allow the brownie to cool on the tray for two hours.
9. Cut the brownie in square pieces.

Oatmeal and Carrot Cake Cookies

Total Prep & Cooking Time: 60 minutes
Yields: 14 Servings
Nutrition Facts: Calories: 94 | Protein: 2.5g | Fat: 2g | Carbs: 15g |
Fiber: 3.6g

Ingredients:

- 100 grams of oats
- 90 grams of flour
- Two tsps. baking powder
- One tsp. cinnamon (ground)
- Half tsp. of salt
- 30 grams of butter (unsalted)
- One egg
- One tsp. of vanilla extract
- 120 ml of maple syrup
- One cup carrot (grated)

Method:

1. Whisk together flour, oats, cinnamon, salt, and baking powder in a bowl.
2. Combine egg, vanilla, and butter in another bowl. Add maple syrup to the mixture.
3. Add the mixture of flour to the mixture of egg. Stir well until combined properly.
4. Add grated carrots.
5. Chill the prepared dough in the freezer for half an hour.
6. Preheat oven at 180 degrees Celsius. Use parchment paper for lining a baking tray.
7. Add the cookie dough to the tray in the form of scoops. Use a spoon for flattening the cookie dough.
8. Bake for fifteen minutes.
9. Cool on the tray for ten minutes.

Choco Chip Cookie Dough

Total Prep & Cooking Time: 40 minutes
Yields: Four Servings
Nutritional Facts: Calories: 221 | Protein: 3g | Fat: 11.1g | Carbs: 36g | Fiber: 5g

Ingredients:

- One tbsp. brown sugar
- Three tbsps. stevia
- Two tbsps. butter
- Five tbsps. flour
- One tsp. salt
- Half tsp. vanilla
- Half tbsp. milk (fat-free)
- Two tbsps. choco chips

Method:

1. Mix sugar, sweetener, and butter in a bowl. Mix until creamy.
2. Add salt, flour, milk, and vanilla. Stir well.
3. Add the chocolate chips to the mix.
4. Chill in the freezer for twenty minutes.

Mango Ice Cream

Total Prep & Cooking Time: 4 hours
Yields: 4 Servings
Nutrition Facts: Calories: 210 | Protein: 6g | Fat: 5g | Carbs: 37g |
Fiber: 1.2g

Ingredients:

- One kg mango (Alphonso)
- 200 grams of milk powder
- 200 ml cream (low-fat)
- One cup milk (skimmed)
- Half cup sugar

Method:

1. Start by peeling the mangoes. Cut the mangoes in cubes.
2. Add the mango cubes in a blender and puree.
3. Add skimmed milk, milk powder, cream, and sugar. Blend again.
4. Pour into a container. Put the container in the freezer for two hours.
5. Beat the ice cream using a fork and put it in the freezer again for two hours.
6. Scoop the ice cream in serving bowls and serve with mango cubes from the top.

Choco Chip and Cherry Ice Cream

Total Prep & Cooking Time: 2 hours
Yields: 4 Servings
Nutrition Facts: Calories: 209 | Protein: 6g | Fat: 5g | Carbs: 21g |
Fiber: 2.3g

Ingredients:

- One can coconut milk
- Two cups cherries (pitted)
- Two tbsps. maple syrup
- Half cup choco chips

Method:

1. Mix one cup cherries, coconut milk, and maple syrup in a blender. Blend the mixture for one minute.
2. Add choco chips and remaining cherries to the mix.
3. Pour the ice cream mix in a container. Put the container in the freezer for two hours.
4. Serve with cherries on top.

Choco Avocado Peanut Butter Pudding

Total Prep & Cooking Time: Two hours and thirty minutes
Yields: Six Servings
Nutrition Facts: Calories: 340 | Protein: 10g | Fat: 27g | Carbs: 25g | Fiber: 612g

Ingredients:

- Two ripe avocados
- One large banana (ripe)
- Half cup cocoa powder (unsweetened)
- One cup peanut butter (crunchy)
- One-fourth cup maple syrup
- One-third cup of almond milk
- Whipped cream (coconut)

Method:

1. Add all the listed ingredients in a food processor except for the cream. Blend the mixture until smooth and creamy.
2. You can add more cocoa powder for a more chocolaty taste.
3. In case you want more sweetness, add maple syrup and blend.
4. Divide the mixture among serving glasses. Cover the glasses with plastic wrap. Chill for two hours in the freezer.
5. Serve with whipped cream on the top.

Roasted Cinnamon and Honey Peaches

Total Prep & Cooking Time: 50 minutes
Yields: Four Servings
Nutritional Facts: Calories: 155 | Protein: 9g | Fat: 2.5g | Carbs: 24g
| Fiber: 2

Ingredients:

- Two tbsp. butter
- Two ripe peaches
- Half tsp. cinnamon (ground)
- Two tbsps. of honey
- Twelve ounces of yogurt (Greek, fat-free)

Method:

1. Preheat the oven at 180 degrees Celsius.
2. Use parchment paper for lining a baking tray.
3. Cut the peaches in half. Remove the peach stones.
4. Top the peaches with half tbsp. butter, half tsp. honey, and cinnamon.
5. Place peaches on the tray. Bake for half an hour.
6. Allow the peaches to cool down.
7. Serve with yogurt by the side.

CHAPTER 8:
7-DAY MEAL PLAN

The Sirtfood Diet has been divided into two phases. The first phase lasts for one week in which you can lose about 7 pounds, according to the developers of the diet. So, in this chapter, you will find a 7-day meal plan for the first phase of the Sirtfood Diet.

Day 1

08:00 AM: Sirtfood Green Juice
12:00 PM: Pineapple Kale Smoothie
04:00 PM: Blueberry Pie Smoothie
08:00 PM: Zucchini Pumpkin Lasagna

Day 2

08:00 AM: Strawberry Smoothie
12:00 PM: Beet Smoothie
04:00 PM: Turmeric Berry Smoothie
08:00 PM: Veggie Coconut Chickpea Curry

Day 3

08:00 AM: Date and blueberry shake
12:00 PM: Avocado blueberry banana smoothie
04:00 PM: Mint avocado smoothie
08:00 PM: Lentil, turmeric, and lemon soup

Day 4

08:00 AM: Kale blueberry smoothie
12:00 PM: Strawberry and chocolate smoothie
04:00 PM: Mixed veggie curry
08:00 PM: Stir-fry chicken satay

Day 5

08:00 AM: Espresso chocolate smoothie
12:00 PM: Mint strawberry smoothie
04:00 PM: Healthy beef chowmein
08:00 PM: Asparagus, noodle, and prawn Salad

Day 6

08:00 AM: Berry banana smoothie
12:00 PM: Berry ginger fruit smoothie
04:00 PM: Healthy chicken korma
08:00 PM: Smoked salmon salad and green dressing

Day 7

08:00 AM: Ginger blueberry peach smoothie
12:00 PM: Mango blueberry smoothie
04:00 PM: Stir-fry hoisin chicken
08:00 PM: Lean pork chops and honey balsamic glaze

CHAPTER 9:
SHOPPING LIST

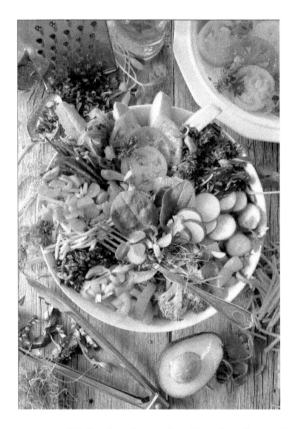

In this chapter, you will find a shopping list for the 7-day meal plan, as given in the previous chapter. Having a well-prepared shopping list in hand will make your shopping task easier, and you will not miss any of the important ingredients.

Fruits

- 1 green apple
- 1 red apple
- 15 bananas
- 1 pineapple

- Blueberries
- Strawberries
- Mixed berries
- 4 avocados
- 1 peach
- 1 ripe mango

Vegetables

- 4 bunches of parsley
- 4 bunches of kale
- 2 stalks of celery
- 2 lemons
- 3 lime
- 40 grams arugula
- 4 gingers
- 1 beet
- 5 bunches of spinach
- 2 bunches of baby spinach
- Mint leaves
- 600 grams butternut pumpkin
- 400 grams pumpkin
- 2 zucchinis
- 7 onions
- 7 garlic
- 5 tomatoes
- 5 cans of tomato
- 3 red onions
- Green chili
- 9 carrots
- 1 Broccoli
- Peas
- 3 bunches of coriander
- 5 stalks of celery
- 400 grams green beans
- 3 potatoes

- 1 cauliflower
- 1 eggplant
- 2 bunches of broccolini
- 2 bunches of pak choy
- 300 grams snow peas
- 450 grams baby corn
- Red chili
- 2 bunches of asparagus
- 3 shallots
- 2 fennel bulbs
- Tarragon
- 1 red capsicum
- 1 yellow capsicum
- 2 spring onions

Starches

- 300grams red lentils
- Chickpeas
- 500 grams quinoa
- 400 grams green lentils

Nuts and Seeds

- Chia seeds
- Flax seed
- Mustard seed
- Sesame seed

Spices and Miscellaneous

- Matcha green tea powder
- Almond milk
- Greek yogurt
- Peanut butter
- Honey
- Almond butter
- Rolled oats

- Vanilla extract
- Cinnamon
- Protein powder
- Maple syrup
- Ground turmeric
- 4 Medjool dates
- Flaxseed meal
- Peppermint extract
- Whipped cream
- Dark chocolate
- Cocoa powder
- Instant espresso coffee
- Coconut milk
- Olive oil
- Allspice
- Oregano
- Ricotta cheese
- Parmesan cheese
- Curry powder
- Vegetable stock
- Curry leaves
- Chili flakes
- Vegetable oil
- Fennel seeds
- Chili powder
- 350 grams chowmein noodles
- Corn flour
- Soy sauce
- Oyster sauce
- Beef stock
- 180 grams soba noodles
- Tamari
- Sesame oil
- Macadamia oil
- 10 cardamom pods
- Chicken stock powder

- Almond meal
- Chives
- Baby capers
- Hoisin sauce
- Peanut oil
- Balsamic vinegar
- Butter
- Rosemary
- Pepper flakes

Fish and Meat

- 500 grams chicken tenderloins
- 500 grams beef mince
- 500 grams prawn
- 900 grams chicken breast
- 180 grams smoked salmon
- 4 pork chops (thick-cut)

CONCLUSION

Thank you for making it through to the end of this book! Let's hope it was informative and able to provide you with all of the tools you need to achieve your goals, whatever they may be.

I hope this book has been able to demonstrate the enormous role that is played by sirtuins in shedding weight. All the basic aspects that help in the functioning of the Sirtfood Diet have been explained. Now, all that you need to do is to start following the diet and promise yourself that you are not going to go off track. The sirtfoods are food items that we use in our kitchen daily. The diet has been divided into different phases, and all that you need to do is follow the phases properly to reap the benefits.

The sirtuins will not only help you to shed weight but will also help in other body functions such as reduction of inflammation. This diet plan is more like a normal lifestyle that you can adopt very easily. It is evident that losing weight cannot be achieved overnight; you will need to wait for it. Consistency is the key to this diet plan, and it will help you to lose a considerable amount of weight within a short time period. I hope you have checked out the 7-day meal plan as it will help you a lot in getting started. You can choose from the wide variety of recipes that have been included in the book to alter the plan.

If you enjoyed this book, please let me know your thoughts by leaving a short review on Amazon. Thank you!

Lightning Source UK Ltd.
Milton Keynes UK
UKHW021851120922
408771UK00003B/75